FUNDAMENTALS OF
NURSING
AND MIDWIFERY
RESEARCH

About the authors

Lisa McKenna (RN RM MEdSt PhD FACN) is Professor and Head in the School of Nursing and Midwifery, La Trobe University, Melbourne. She has researched widely, particularly in the areas of nursing, midwifery and health professional education and workforce, and published over 170 refereed peer reviewed journal articles along with a number of textbooks. Lisa's research expertise incorporates a range of methodologies, including quantitative, qualitative and mixed methods, and she has supervised many honours, masters and doctoral projects to successful completion. Lisa is also Editor-in-Chief of *Collegian: The Australian Journal of Nursing Practice, Scholarship and Research*.

Beverley Copnell (RN BAppSc PhD) is Associate Professor in the School of Nursing and Midwifery, La Trobe University, Melbourne. Before entering academia, she worked for many years in paediatric intensive care, a field in which she maintains an active interest. She served two terms as a member of the Board of Directors of the World Federation of Paediatric Intensive and Critical Care Societies (2003–2011) and is a member of the editorial board of *Pediatric Critical Care Medicine*. She has published widely on a range of topics in this and other fields. She has a long-standing interest in promoting research and evidence-based practice in nursing, and has taught related subjects at both undergraduate and postgraduate levels. She is an editor of *Collegian: The Australian Journal of Nursing Practice, Scholarship and Research*.

LISA McKENNA | BEVERLEY COPNELL

FUNDAMENTALS OF
NURSING AND
MIDWIFERY RESEARCH

A practical guide for evidence-based practice

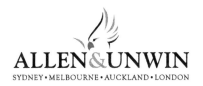

ALLEN&UNWIN
SYDNEY·MELBOURNE·AUCKLAND·LONDON

Allen & Unwin
83 Alexander Street
Crows Nest NSW 2065
Australia
Phone: (61 2) 8425 0100
Email: info@allenandunwin.com
Web: www.allenandunwin.com

 A catalogue record for this
book is available from the
National Library of Australia

ISBN 978 1 76063 109 3

Type design by Squirt Creative
Set in 11/15 pt Legacy Serif ITC by Midland Typesetters, Australia
Printed and bound in Australia by SOS Print + Media Group

10 9 8 7 6 5 4 3 2 1

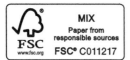 The paper in this book is FSC® certified.
FSC® promotes environmentally responsible,
socially beneficial and economically viable
management of the world's forests.

CONTENTS

DETAILED CONTENTS

Chapter 4   Understanding quantitative research approaches 57

Chapter 5   Understanding qualitative research approaches 89

LIST OF FIGURES AND TABLES

FIGURES

TABLES

LIST OF BOXES

RESEARCH EXAMPLES

RESEARCH TIPS

ACTIVITIES

OUTLINE OF THE BOOK

SECTION 1 HOW DO I FIND AND USE EVIDENCE?

Chapter 1 provides an introduction to evidence in nursing and midwifery. The chapter discusses the importance of using evidence in practice and outcomes when health professionals do not use evidence to support their practice. It positions research in the context of evidence and outlines the need for nurses and midwives to be users of evidence. It uses Nursing and Midwifery Board of Australia standards to reinforce its importance.

Chapter 2 provides a focus on locating evidence to support nursing and midwifery practice. The chapter examines sources of research evidence along with strategies for effectively finding it and determining its credibility. It presents common databases where nursing and midwifery research can be found, and strategies for conducting effective searches within them.

SECTION 2 HOW CAN I MAKE SENSE OF RESEARCH EVIDENCE?

Chapter 3 provides an overview of various steps involved in the research process. It introduces considerations in developing a research question, deciding the best approach for a research study, designing a study, and identifying and accessing necessary approvals.

Chapter 4 provides an overview of quantitative research approaches commonly used in nursing and midwifery, with a focus on person-centred care. The chapter examines experimental and non-experimental research designs, and processes for developing a quantitative research question. It explores different types of data, sampling procedures, data collection, basic statistical tests and the importance of validity and reliability. Finally, it discusses reporting of quantitative findings and related reporting standards.

Chapter 5 provides an overview of qualitative research approaches commonly used in nursing and midwifery, with a focus on person-centred care. The chapter explores reasons why qualitative research is popular in nursing and midwifery and introduces common approaches—namely, phenomenology, descriptive qualitative approaches and grounded theory. Using a case study, it explores steps in undertaking qualitative research, common data collection methods, sampling approaches and analysing qualitative data using thematic and content analysis. Finally, it examines considerations for ensuring the quality of qualitative research, and reporting findings.

SECTION 3 HOW DO I CRITICALLY EVALUATE RESEARCH STUDIES?

Chapter 6 provides an overview of processes for critiquing research. It introduces a step-by-step approach to evaluating research quality through questioning and critiquing tools. Using the case example of vital signs monitoring, the chapter examines the value of nursing and midwifery research. It introduces the collation of research critiques of bodies of knowledge to explore approaches to structured critical literature reviews—namely, systematic and scoping reviews—including protocol development.

Chapter 7 provides an overview of ethical considerations in nursing and midwifery research. The chapter introduces the importance of ethical approaches to research and the roles of Human Research Ethics Committees. It presents a range of fundamental principles that should underpin all research involving human participants, including research merit and integrity, beneficence and non-maleficence, respect for persons and justice. Finally, the chapter explores ethical issues arising in the emerging use of the internet and social media as data sources in research.

SECTION 4 HOW DO I USE RESEARCH EVIDENCE TO INFORM MY PRACTICE?

Chapter 8 provides an overview of approaches to applying research evidence to nursing and midwifery practice. The chapter introduces the concept of knowledge translation and the questioning of clinical practice. It presents clinical practice guidelines and clinical audits as sources of practice evidence. The chapter examines some common evidence-based practice models used in health care. Finally, it explores evaluation of evidence implementation using action research and realist evaluation as sample approaches.

Chapter 9 is dedicated to the writing of effective reviews of the literature. The chapter begins by defining what a literature review seeks to achieve, types of literature reviews and the process of writing a review. It introduces a range of academic concepts important to students needing to undertake reviews of literature for academic assessments as well as for clinical work.

SECTION 5 HOW DO I PURSUE A NURSING OR MIDWIFERY RESEARCH FUTURE?

Chapter 10 provides insights into research career pathways available to nurses and midwives. It introduces different types of research roles common to these professions and education pathways to research careers. The second half of the chapter focuses on seeking funding for research activities and developing effective proposals for grant funding or academic work.

PREFACE

In today's contemporary healthcare system, research plays a major role in directing the best approaches to clinical care and practice. This is no different for the disciplines of nursing and midwifery, where increasingly there is an onus to provide the most effective care, informed by quality and current research findings. Consumers of health care, too, are much better informed than they have been in the past. With access to endless online information resources, they expect the highest levels of treatments and care. Thus, the concept of evidence-based care has to become central to the practice of nurses and midwives.

Over past decades, nurses and midwives have cared for patients based upon traditional knowledge and practices. Many have continued to practise in the ways they were originally taught in their pre-registration courses. However, this is no longer appropriate. Nurses and midwives have a professional responsibility to keep up-to-date with current research impacting on their clinical practice. This occurs in a context where there is increasing emphasis on research and rapid growth in the production of research by nurses, midwives and other health professionals. Nurses and midwives require the skills and knowledge to read and understand research reports, evaluate the quality of the research, synthesise different research studies, apply the most appropriate findings to their clinical practice and evaluate their effectiveness. Furthermore, many nurses and midwives desire to contribute directly to the production of relevant research, requiring skills in performing quality research studies relevant to their practice.

We have written this text to be a useful introduction to research and evidence-based practice for nursing and midwifery students and clinicians. It aims to be practical in its approach, so that it can be used across various stages of the professional's career. We hope to demystify the connection between research and practice for students and clinicians. Each chapter in the book has been written with an overarching case study, allowing introduced concepts to be applied to realistic situations and made less distant from clinical practice. These concepts have been kept simple to ensure they are relevant, even to the beginning student of nursing or midwifery. In each chapter, we have also presented examples of actual research studies that have been conducted and are relevant to the topic being covered to demonstrate examples of how these aspects have been studied. Throughout each chapter, we include a number of activities to assist the learner to work directly with concepts as they apply to their individual situation. At the end of each chapter, we have included a series of review and reflection questions to facilitate assessment of learning and understanding, as well as questions that can be used to promote discussions in research groups or class-based situations.

The text has been developed as a series of sections that aim to progressively build the reader's fundamental knowledge and skills. Section 1 consists of two chapters. Within this section, Chapter 1 introduces the concept of evidence and explains why nurses and midwives need to understand research. The chapter introduces various professional and regulatory requirements for nurses and midwives to use evidence-based practice. Chapter 2 begins to explore how and where relevant evidence can be found, facilitating skills in searching for evidence.

Section 2 is focused on making sense of research evidence. This section contains three chapters that give an overview of research and different research approaches to provide a foundation for the reader in reading and understanding a variety of types of research studies. Chapter 3 presents a detailed introduction to the research process and how one goes about doing a research study. Chapter 4 examines quantitative research approaches with an overview of types of studies and statistical tests. Chapter 5 explores a variety of qualitative approaches to research, including how they can be undertaken.

Section 3 focuses on assisting the reader to develop skills in critically reading and evaluating research that could be used to inform clinical practice. This section consists of two chapters. Chapter 6 details step-by-step approaches to evaluating the quality of research studies and their applicability to practice. Chapter 7 introduces the important area of ethics in research. It provides an overview of ethical processes and considerations underpinning the conduct of research, ensuring that the reader has the skills to evaluate whether research has been conducted ethically.

Section 4 takes the learning from previous chapters into its application through evidence-based practice. This section consists of two chapters. Chapter 8 examines the concept of knowledge translation and how evidence can be taken from published research into guiding clinical practice. The important aspect of evaluating the application of research evidence to practice is detailed in this chapter. Chapter 9 builds on previous chapters to examine how research can be synthesised into different types of literature reviews to inform and guide practice.

In a context where nurses and midwives are increasingly engaging in research activity, the final section, consisting of one chapter, explores potential research career pathways. Chapter 10 examines the nurse or midwife as evidence generator, as well as research roles that nurses and midwives assume. The chapter examines available educational pathways that can be taken to further develop research expertise. Increasingly, nurses and midwives are expected to write proposals for research, whether for educational purposes or when seeking funding to support their research ideas. The chapter concludes with a step-by-step overview of how to go about writing an effective research proposal and suggests avenues that can be pursued for seeking funding to support research.

We hope that students and clinicians alike will find this text to be a valuable resource, assisting them to understand research and its application to clinical nursing and midwifery practice and contributing to the delivery of up-to-date and relevant evidence-informed optimal care.

Lisa McKenna
Beverley Copnell

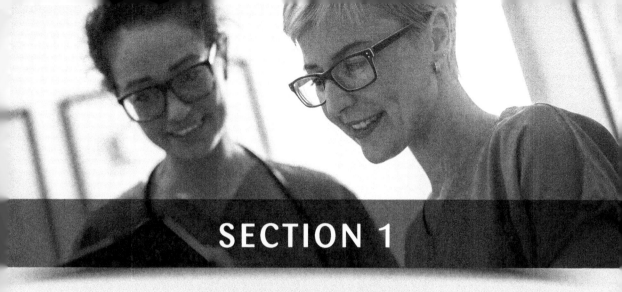

SECTION 1

HOW DO I FIND
AND USE EVIDENCE?

Evidence-based practice is a key requirement of the work of nurses and midwives. It is mandated as a part of competency standards and works to ensure the care delivered to patients is based on research proving its effectiveness. It is not considered appropriate for nurses and midwives to continue to practise in the same way throughout their careers; rather, practice needs to develop according to new and emerging research. Furthermore, today's healthcare consumers are more educated than in past decades. Through the internet, people have ready access to up-to-date research findings and are more informed about their conditions and expectations of care. This increases the requirement for nurses and midwives to be abreast of current evidence relevant to their daily practice.

This section is dedicated to the area of evidence for nursing and midwifery practice. It examines the professional requirements for incorporating evidence into practice. Through a particular focus on hand hygiene, the section examines what constitutes evidence, locating appropriate evidence and evidence appraisal.

Chapter 1 introduces the concept of evidence and why it is important for nursing and midwifery. It explores what it means to be a user of evidence and introduces hierarchies of evidence.

Chapter 2 builds on the previous chapter to examine where and how credible evidence can be found, and the appraisal of evidence for informing practice.

CHAPTER 1

What is evidence and why do I need to understand research?

LEARNING OBJECTIVES

After working through this chapter, you should be able to:

- discuss what is meant by *evidence* in nursing and midwifery
- outline the importance of evidence for health professional practice
- discuss the relationship between evidence and research in nursing and midwifery
- identify the role of the nurse or midwife as a user of evidence
- define the term *evidence-based practice*
- identify sources of good evidence
- outline professional requirements for nurses and midwives in relation to evidence-based practice
- define the term *systematic review.*

KEY TERMS AND CONCEPTS

Data analysis, data collection, dissemination, evidence, evidence-based practice, hierarchy of evidence, hypothesis, literature review, practice guidelines, research, research process, research question, quality patient care, systematic review

CASE STUDY OVERVIEW

Effective handwashing is an important, and sometimes underestimated, task of health professionals that has the potential to directly impact on the wellbeing of patients. If micro-organisms are allowed to move from person to person through poor handwashing, this can result in serious nosocomial (hospital-acquired) infections, which may require prolonged hospitalisation or even lead to unintended deaths. Effective handwashing is, therefore, fundamentally important. However, varying advice exists about correct handwashing techniques and for how long handwashing should take place. In addition, hospitals provide alcohol-based disinfectants for hand sanitisation. How then do health professionals know the most effective methods of hand hygiene to reduce negative patient outcomes?

CHAPTER INTRODUCTION

Evidence-based practice is a key requirement of the work of nurses and midwives. Hence, an understanding of evidence and how it informs practice is important. This chapter introduces the concept of evidence in nursing and midwifery and how this evidence relates to practice. It also clarifies the connection between evidence and research and its importance in evidence-based nursing practice. Hierarchies of evidence are discussed, along with the role of systematic review and its benefits for nursing and midwifery.

What is evidence?

Nursing and midwifery practice is described as being underpinned by **evidence**. However, what does that mean? Using our case study about handwashing, we can begin to define it. The case study raises a question about how health professionals know the most effective methods of hand hygiene to reduce negative patient outcomes. This is where evidence comes in. Evidence in such cases relates to research findings that inform the best possible practice. Take, for example, a 2015 study conducted to compare the effectiveness of alcohol-based disinfectants with that of handwashing with soap and water in reducing the spread of different viruses. Washing hands with soap and water for 30 seconds was found to be more effective than using the alcohol-based products in removing norovirus, a virus that often causes gastroenteritis outbreaks in nursing homes (Tuladhar et al. 2015). This suggests that in some practice settings handwashing for 30 seconds with soap and water is the most effective option; hence, such evidence should guide practice.

evidence
knowledge derived from systematic research

So, going back to our original question, evidence is information, generated through research, that supports nursing and midwifery practice. In some cases, the findings from many research studies have been collated into practice guidelines that can directly inform health professionals' practice. The extent of infection acquired through hand contact led the World Health Organization to use evidence to develop its own practice guidelines for use across Australian health care. This led to the creation of the Five Moments for Hand Hygiene. Using research findings, five key moments when microorganisms can spread via hand contact in health care were identified:

1   Before patient contact
2   Before aseptic task
3   After body fluid exposure risk
4   After patient contact
5   After contact with patient surroundings. (World Health Organization 2017)

This process has been adopted by the Australian Commission on Safety and Quality in Health Care (2017) as part of the National Hand Hygiene Initiative to reduce nosocomial infection, so it directly impacts on the practice of health professionals in Australia. Practice guidelines such as these also constitute evidence for practice, as they have been developed based upon the collation of findings of rigorous research.

What happens if health professionals do not use evidence?

Quality health care is dependent on health professionals applying current evidence to support the care they deliver to patients and communities. However, many health professionals do not adopt new practice supported by the latest evidence, choosing instead to continue with the practice they were originally taught. While that practice was probably seen to be the most effective at the time they learnt it, it may since have been disproven by research. In such cases, patients may receive inappropriate or ineffective care or may be put at increased risk of complications. If we take hand hygiene and the research by Tuladhar et al. (2015) as an example, a health professional who is carrying norovirus and washes their hands for 10 seconds may carry the virus on to the next patient, who may subsequently become infected and develop gastroenteritis, which can have very serious consequences for the elderly and frail. Hence, evidence that directly informs practice can enhance patient care and health outcomes.

ACTIVITY 1.1 Evidence in nursing and midwifery practice

List the key reasons why nurses and midwives need to use evidence in practice.

Where does research fit in?

So far, we have explored the role of evidence in nursing and midwifery practice and alluded to its connection with research. However, just collecting existing research is not sufficient to implement it into practice. There is good research and not-so-good research, so it is important to understand the **research process** and to critique or evaluate the quality of the research in order to determine whether or not to use it to support practice.

research process
the whole process of conducting research, from the original idea to the dissemination of findings

In this section of the chapter, we will begin to explore the research process, and we will continue to build on this in subsequent chapters.

While there are various approaches to research, all follow a consistent and systematic process:

- **Problem or issue** Generally, research is conducted to generate new knowledge to address a particular problem or examine an issue.
- **Literature review** Existing research studies are explored to see if the problem has already been addressed. If the research has already been done, there may be no need for new studies to be conducted. However,

if there is a gap in the existing literature, it is an indication for new research to be conducted. Hence, the literature review provides the background against which a new study is developed.

- **Research question** From the problem or issue, the researcher develops a question—the research question—which the research seeks to answer. The research question should be clear, specific and able to be answered.

- **Ethical approval** If the study requires the collection of data relating to humans or animals, the researcher will be required to have the work evaluated by an ethics committee to ensure it is to be conducted in an ethical manner. The aim of ethical consideration is to confirm that the participants' rights are adhered to and participants are not put at any unnecessary risk by taking part in the research.

- **Data collection** The researcher next determines the best way, or method, in which to collect the data needed to answer the research question. This can take a number of forms—for example, questionnaires, interviews or observations.

- **Data analysis** Once all of the data are collected, the researcher analyses them to determine the research findings. This might involve mathematical calculations for numerical data or identification of patterns of words or phrases for text-based data.

- **Reporting or dissemination** Once the findings have been determined, they are made available for others to apply them. Study findings are often reported through published peer-reviewed journal articles and at professional conferences, or may be presented directly in reports to governments or other organisations.

We will explore these steps in more detail in Chapter 3.

Being a user of research

Nurses and midwives are increasingly undertaking research to add to the evidence base and improve the care they deliver. However, while not all will actually undertake research, all nurses and midwives are required to use research to underpin their practice, as any other professional does.

This is reinforced through the Nursing and Midwifery Board of Australia's professional practice standards for the disciplines:

- **Registered Nurse Standards for Practice** says that registered nurses 'use a variety of thinking strategies and the best available evidence in making decisions and providing safe, quality nursing practice within person-centred and evidence-based frameworks'. The standard also states that the registered nurse 'accesses, analyses, and uses the best available evidence, that includes research findings, for safe, quality practice' (NMBA 2016, Standard 1.1).

- **National Competency Standards for the Midwife** establishes the midwife's responsibility to use research to inform practice, stating that the midwife 'ensures research evidence is incorporated into practice' and 'interprets evidence as a basis to inform practice and decision making' (NMBA 2006, Competency 14.1–2).

RESEARCH EXAMPLE 1.1 Hand hygiene practices

Hand hygiene is fundamental to prevention of the spread of infection. Exploring hand hygiene practices assists with identifying issues that may impact on their effectiveness and on the wellbeing of patients. Castle et al. (2016) developed a questionnaire to explore the opinions of nurse aides working in nursing homes across the United States about their hand hygiene practices. They received data from 4211 nurse aides working in 767 nursing homes. The researchers found that 57.4 per cent complied with hand-washing most of the time when caring for clients, with only 21.7 per cent reporting they always complied. Within the nursing homes studied, only 43.3 per cent reported checking that handwashing was occurring.

N. Castle, S. Handler & L. Wagner, 2016, 'Hand hygiene practices reported by nurse aides in nursing homes', *Journal of Applied Gerontology*, vol. 35, no. 3, pp. 267–285.

Questions for consideration
- What are the implications of this study's findings?
- How might nurses use this evidence to improve care?

The standards' requirements for nurses and midwives to practise in an evidence-based way serve to ensure that patients and other health consumers receive the most effective care informed by best practice. They also serve to protect nurses and midwives, by making them accountable for their practice and the care they deliver should they be questioned about their actions in any particular situation.

As a mandated component of the roles of nurses and midwives, evidence needs to be translated directly into practice. However, research into this area suggests that it can be challenging. A cross-sectional survey (see Chapter 4) conducted by Stokke et al. (2014) in Norway with 185 nurses found that nurses held positive views about **evidence-based practice**; however, they only practised it to a small extent. This was attributed to their feeling unprepared to undertake evidence-based practice and their belief that resources to do so were limited. The researchers concluded that it was important to be educationally prepared to use evidence and that there was a need for a culture in the clinical setting to facilitate it.

evidence-based practice
practice informed by best available research evidence, clinical expertise and client preference

---

RESEARCH EXAMPLE 1.2 Barriers in evidence-based nursing practice

While evidence-based practice is recognised as vital for effective patient care, nurses have been slow to adopt it. Many studies have explored nurses' use of research in practice to attempt to understand why this is the case. In one study, Hendricks and Cope (2017) sought to discover whether nurses read research articles, understood them and used the findings in practice. The researchers used a survey of nurses in one hospital in Western Australia. A total of 95 nurses completed the survey. The findings indicated that the nurses found research articles difficult to understand, and 84 per cent reported only sometimes understanding what they were reading. In addition, 64 per cent had not taken any studies in research. This reinforces the need for nurses to have the skills to interpret research findings.

J. Hendricks & V. Cope, 2017, 'Research is not a "scary" word: Registered nurses and the barriers to research utilisation', *Nordic Journal of Nursing Research*, vol. 37, no. 1, pp. 44–50.

Questions for consideration

- Do you think the findings of this study are common to all nurses and midwives?
- What strategies could be used to develop necessary skills for reading and understanding research in nurses and midwives?

RESEARCH EXAMPLE 1.3 Evidence-based practice in midwifery

Little has been written about midwives' application of research findings to their care of childbearing women. However, evidence-based practice is key to ensuring women receive the most effective and appropriate care. In one US study, Kennedy et al. (2012) conducted research to understand midwives' perspectives on evidence-based practice and how an organised network could assist their work. They undertook interviews with 23 nurse-midwives. Their findings indicated that there were numerous challenges to implementing evidence-based practice within their workplaces from people with influence. The participants found it difficult to challenge existing practices, even if the evidence did not support them, but they worked to keep up-to-date with recent literature and to influence change when they could. One particular reported challenge emerged when women requested to have interventions that were not evidence based.

H.P. Kennedy, E. Doig, B. Hackley & M.S. Leslie, 2012, '"The midwifery two-step": A study on evidence-based midwifery practice', *Journal of Midwifery and Women's Health*, vol. 57, pp. 454–460.

Questions for consideration

- Do you think the findings of this study are common to all nurses and midwives?
- How might nurses and midwives manage requests for interventions that are not evidence based?

Determining levels of evidence

Not all research is considered equal. Evidence elicited from some types of research is regarded as being more credible than others, and evidence sources are ranked into a hierarchy. In the National Health and Medical

Research Council **hierarchy of evidence**, the highest level is accorded to systematic reviews of randomised controlled trials (NHMRC 2009). While we will not delve into the various types of studies in detail here, it is important to

hierarchy of evidence
levels of authority attributed to different forms of research evidence

acknowledge that there are different types of evidence and that these are accorded varied levels of credibility.

Systematic review

At the top of the National Health and Medical Research Council's hierarchy of evidence sits systematic review of randomised controlled trials (see Chapter 4). A **systematic review** is an analysis of a collection of

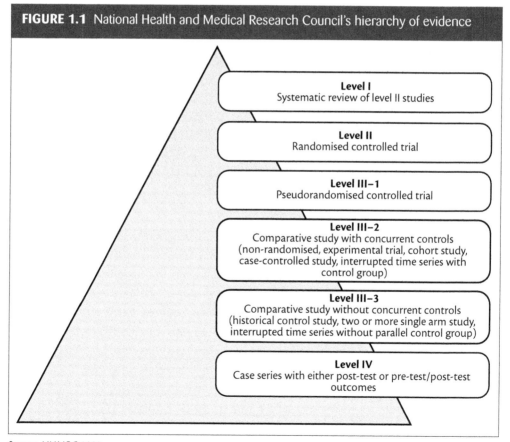

FIGURE 1.1 National Health and Medical Research Council's hierarchy of evidence

Level I
Systematic review of level II studies

Level II
Randomised controlled trial

Level III–1
Pseudorandomised controlled trial

Level III–2
Comparative study with concurrent controls
(non-randomised, experimental trial, cohort study,
case-controlled study, interrupted time series with
control group)

Level III–3
Comparative study without concurrent controls
(historical control study, two or more single arm study,
interrupted time series without parallel control group)

Level IV
Case series with either post-test or pre-test/post-test
outcomes

Source: NHMRC 2009

systematic review
a literature review that uses a structured question and search approach along with critical appraisal and quality analysis of studies

individual studies on the same topic that is conducted in a structured and auditable way. In a sense, systematic reviews are research studies in their own right. These types of reviews are becoming an increasingly popular undertaking with nurses and midwives. One reason for this is that they collate the findings of smaller research studies to draw larger conclusions, and much of the research conducted by nurses and midwives is small and local in nature, unlike that in other scientific disciplines. Often, systematic reviews are also used to identify gaps in existing knowledge, to guide development of new studies.

Similar to a research study, a systematic review is underpinned by a specific question or aim. To demonstrate, we will examine a systematic review conducted by Huis et al. (2012) that sought to explore the effectiveness of strategies to increase hand hygiene compliance. The researchers sought to identify frequently used strategies for compliance and the related determinants of behaviour change that led to positive hand hygiene behaviour.

The next step in systematic review is to develop a protocol (outline) defining the boundaries and inclusion criteria for the review—for example, which databases will be searched, the timeframe from which papers will be included, the type of study design that will be used, the population that will be studied and the keywords and phrases that will be used to undertake the search for relevant studies. Huis et al. (2012) included experimental and quasi-experimental research (see Chapter 4) from January 2000 to November 2009. They searched a number of databases, including MEDLINE, Embase, CINAHL and Cochrane. From this, they identified 119 studies as potentially meeting their inclusion criteria and on closer examination found a total of 41 to be included for analysis. Many were excluded because the research was considered to be of poor quality. A key aspect of systematic review is assessment of the quality of each study according to set evaluation criteria.

Once the final papers for inclusion have been determined, they can be grouped for analysis. Examination of the final 41 papers used in the review by Huis et al. (2012) demonstrated that there were hidden and valuable components embedded within hand hygiene strategies. They concluded that addressing just some aspects, such as knowledge and awareness, was not sufficient to improve hand hygiene practices; rather, a combination of factors at the levels of individual clinician, team and the organisation needed to be considered. These findings have the potential to influence educators developing programs for improving hand hygiene compliance.

RESEARCH EXAMPLE 1.4 A systematic review of hand hygiene practices

In 2015, Luangasanatip et al. published a systematic review of 41 research studies. They sought to evaluate the effectiveness of the World Health Organization's hand hygiene campaign that commenced in 2005. The findings suggested that the program had been effective at increasing hand hygiene compliance in healthcare workers. They also concluded that further improvements could be achieved by setting goals, putting incentives in place and improving accountability. Furthermore, they concluded that the reporting of resources needed to promote hand hygiene was not adequate.

N. Luangasanatip, M. Hongsuwan, D. Limmathurotsakul, Y. Lubell, A.S. Lee, S. Harbarth, N.P.J. Day, N. Graves, B.S. Cooper, 2015, 'Comparative efficacy of interventions to promote hand hygiene in hospital: Systematic review and network meta-analysis', *British Medical Journal*, vol. 351, article h3728.

Questions for consideration
- How might nurses and midwives put these findings into practice?
- What is the benefit of collating studies in a systematic review?

CHAPTER SUMMARY

Evidence is fundamental to effective nursing and midwifery practice. This chapter has introduced the concept of evidence and the importance of reliable evidence for quality care delivery. The relationship between evidence and research has been discussed, along with an overview of the research process. The responsibility of nurses and midwives to be research utilisers has been considered. Finally, hierarchies of evidence have been introduced, with a focus on systematic review.

In the next chapter, we will build on this work to examine processes for finding suitable evidence and assessing its quality.

CHAPTER REVIEW QUESTIONS

- What is meant by *evidence* in nursing and midwifery practice?
- What is the relationship between evidence and research?
- What professional requirements impact on nurses' and midwives' use of evidence in practice?
- What are the key steps in the research process?
- What constitutes a systematic review?

QUESTIONS FOR DISCUSSION

- Why is evidence important for nursing, midwifery and health professional practice?
- How can nurses and midwives contribute to research knowledge and use?
- What are some of the challenges nurses and midwives face in utilising evidence in practice?
- What strategies could be used to promote evidence application in nursing and midwifery practice?

QUESTIONS FOR PERSONAL REFLECTION

- What are your personal expectations of healthcare providers with regard to being abreast of current evidence in their field?
- What strategies can you employ to build your understanding of evidence and research in your own profession?
- How do you see your own professional responsibilities with regard to evidence-based practice?

USEFUL WEB RESOURCES

Australian Nursing and Midwifery Federation's research policy <http://anf.org.au/documents/policies/P_Nursing_Midwifery_Research.pdf>

National Health and Medical Research Council on research <www.nhmrc.gov.au/research>

National Institute of Nursing Research (United States) <www.ninr.nih.gov>

REFERENCES AND FURTHER READING

Australian Commission on Safety and Quality in Health Care, 2017, *National Hand Hygiene Initiative*, <www.safetyandquality.gov.au/our-work/healthcare-associated-infection/hand-hygiene/>.

Castle, N., Handler, S. & Wagner, L., 2016, 'Hand hygiene practices reported by nurse aides in nursing homes', *Journal of Applied Gerontology*, vol. 35, no. 3, pp. 267–285.

Hendricks, J. & Cope, V., 2017, 'Research is not a "scary" word: Registered nurses and the barriers to research utilisation', *Nordic Journal of Nursing Research*, vol. 37, no. 1, pp. 44–50.

Huis, A., van Achterberg, T., de Bruin, M., Grol, R., Schoonhoven, L. & Hulscher, M., 2012, 'A systematic review of hand hygiene improvement strategies: A behavioural approach', *Implementation Science*, vol. 7, article 92, <www.implementationscience.com/content/7/1/92>.

Kennedy, H.P., Doig, E., Hackley B. & Leslie, M.S., 2012, '"The midwifery two-step": A study on evidence-based midwifery practice', *Journal of Midwifery and Women's Health*, vol. 57, pp. 454–460.

Luangasanatip, N., Hongsuwan, M., Limmathurotsakul, D., Lubell, Y., Lee, A.S., Harbarth, S., Day, N.P.J., Graves, N. & Cooper, B.S., 2015, 'Comparative efficacy of interventions to promote hand hygiene in hospital: Systematic review and network meta-analysis', *British Medical Journal*, vol. 351, article h3728.

National Health and Medical Research Council *see* NHMRC

NHMRC, 2009, *NHMRC Levels of Evidence and Grades for Recommendations for Developers of Guidelines*, <www.nhmrc.gov.au/_files_nhmrc/file/guidelines/developers/nhmrc_levels_grades_evidence_120423.pdf>.

NMBA, 2006, *National Competency Standards for the Midwife*, NMBA, Melbourne.

NMBA, 2016, *Registered Nurse Standards for Practice*, NMBA, Melbourne.

Nursing and Midwifery Board of Australia *see* NMBA

Stokke, K., Olsen, N.R., Espehaug, B. & Nortvedt, M.W., 2014, 'Evidence based practice beliefs and implementation among nurses: A cross-sectional study', *BMC Nursing*, vol. 13, no. 8, <www.biomedcentral.com/1472-6955/13/8>.

Tuladhar, E., Hazeleger, W.C., Koopmans, M., Zwietering, M.H., Duizer, H. & Beumer, R.R., 2015, 'Reducing viral contamination from finger pads: Handwashing is more effective than alcohol-based hand disinfectants', *Journal of Hospital Infection*, vol. 90, no. 3, pp. 226–234.

World Health Organization, 2017, *Five Moments for Hand Hygiene*, <http://who.int/gpsc/tools/Five_moments/en/>.

CHAPTER 2

Locating evidence

LEARNING OBJECTIVES

After working through this chapter, you should be able to:

- discuss different types of evidence used to support nursing and midwifery practice
- identify credible sources of evidence
- search for and locate appropriate literature to help answer a clinical question
- utilise a variety of academic databases containing nursing and midwifery research
- construct effective evidence searching strategies
- differentiate between levels of evidence in various types of research.

KEY TERMS AND CONCEPTS

Boolean operator, databases, evidence, evidence hierarchies, journals, keywords, levels of evidence, Medical Subject Headings, MeSH terms, truncator, wildcard

CASE STUDY OVERVIEW

For a university assignment, Laura is required to find and summarise evidence on a particular aspect of handwashing. The assignment instructions state that the evidence must be no more than five years old and must be relevant to nurses. Students can choose which aspect they focus on. Laura decides to look at barriers to handwashing.

CHAPTER INTRODUCTION

The previous chapter introduced the concept of evidence-based practice and its import-ance in nursing. Evidence in this context is defined as knowledge derived from systematic research. This chapter examines sources of existing research evidence and describes how to undertake a search for evidence. Evidence hierarchies, introduced in the previous chapter, are explored in more detail.

Where can I find evidence?

When we talk about looking for information, whether for an assignment, a literature review or any other reason, it is important to distinguish between research evidence and other types of information that are not derived from research. The latter may be useful (for instance, in provid-ing background or contextual information) but do not directly address the specific topic or question. Finding evidence means finding reports of completed research. While there is a wide range of sources of general information, not all of these are useful in locating evidence.

The most useful source of reported research is academic journals, in which research is published in the form of articles, or papers. Journals may be discipline specific (for example, nursing, midwifery, medical, allied health disciplines), speciality specific (for example, paediatric, mental health, oncology) or both. Journals are not all of the same quality; in Chapter 6 we will look at how to evaluate a journal to assist in deciding how credible the evidence is. Research published in repu-table journals has been subjected to a process called **peer review**, which means it has been evaluated by at least two people who are likely to have expertise in the area of research, the methods used or both. The article will have been through a number of changes before the review-ers and the editor of the journal were confident that it was fit to publish. Sometimes very large studies are published in book form because there is too much information to fit in to the confines of a journal article. The book will usually have undergone a review of some kind, but the process may not be clear to a reader. Textbooks, a common

peer review
the process of evaluating an article for its suitability for publication. It is usually undertaken by a minimum of two people with expertise in the topic, the methods used, or both

source of information for student assignments, are unlikely to contain research reports, although they may include references to research, which can be used to find original reports. However, as textbooks take some time to write and publish, the references may not reflect the latest research findings.

Research reports can sometimes be found outside academic sources, in which case they are said to be **grey literature**. There are several reasons why research findings may not be published in journals or books. The research may have been completed very recently and the researchers have only presented it at a conference, in which case the **abstract** (or sometimes the whole presentation) will have been published in the conference proceedings. The research may have been undertaken by government or other institutions and disseminated only as a standalone report. It may have been carried out as part of a university higher degree and written up only as a thesis. These types of research reports may not have been subjected to the same scrutiny as academic journal articles, and therefore their credibility can be questionable.

grey literature
literature not published in academic sources

abstract
a summary of a published article or a conference presentation

Table 2.1 lists commonly used sources of information, their usefulness in terms of locating research evidence, and their credibility. Academic journals are the best and most useful sources of research evidence. However, journals publish several types of articles in addition to research reports—for instance, editorials, letters, and discussion and opinion pieces. These kinds of articles are not considered evidence; therefore, it is important to be able to recognise the different categories. Many journals actually indicate the category within the article itself, so this is the first thing to look for. Reports of research studies are characterised by the following:

- They usually include the word *research* or *study* somewhere in the abstract or in the early part of the article.
- They give a clearly expressed aim, usually at the end of the introduction section, which makes it clear that the article is reporting on a research study.

- They include a section labelled 'Methods' or 'Methodology', and the study design (see Section 2) should be obvious. Many journals, but not all, insist that the design is specified in the article title.
- They have a section called 'Results' or 'Findings'.

Another type of article, which may have a similar format to that listed above, is a literature review, which brings together some or all of the literature on a particular topic. There are different kinds of review articles; we will look at these in detail in Chapters 8 and 9. They can be useful when beginning to explore a topic, as they can help clarify ideas, they quickly give an overview of the sort of research that has been done on the topic, and their reference lists can help to find original research reports. However, they are not usually considered evidence in themselves. An exception is a specific type of literature review called a *systematic review* (introduced in

TABLE 2.1 Information sources and their usefulness and credibility as sources of research evidence

Source	Availability of evidence	Accessibility of evidence	Credibility
Journals	The commonest location	Easy to find	High
Books	Relatively rare	Can be difficult to find	Probably good; may not be clear
Textbooks	Unlikely to find	N/A	Probably good; may not be clear
Theses	Common location	Can be difficult to find	Unclear
Websites	Sometimes can be found	Full report may not be available	Unclear; not recommended except in specific circumstances
Mass media, social media	Findings may be mentioned	Full report not available	Unclear; locate original source

Chapter 1), which is carried out using a highly rigorous process and aims to reanalyse the findings of the included studies. Literature review articles should be identified as such in the title, the abstract or both.

How do I find evidence?

Although some print versions are produced, most journals nowadays are published online, which simplifies finding and retrieving their content. However, it is neither efficient nor effective to attempt to find literature by using a generic search engine, such as Google. First, search engines do not have the ability to perform complex search procedures that eliminate irrelevant material at the same time as finding relevant material that may use slightly different terminology from your search term. Second, as most journals require a subscription, you will be unable to retrieve most of the articles you find in this way. Lastly, it can be very difficult for inexperienced researchers to discern the quality of the results returned by search engines.

Journal articles can be found using a specifically targeted search engine such as Google Scholar, and you can be more confident in the quality of the material found by this type of search engine. However, the other limitations still apply. Usually, these search engines are used only in specific circumstances (for example, when undertaking a systematic review; see Chapter 6) to ensure no articles have been missed.

The best way to find research evidence is by searching a database—an electronic catalogue, or index. When you search a database, you are not searching the internet. There are hundreds of commercially available databases (and a few that are publicly available) that can be accessed through hospital and university libraries. Most databases are discipline specific, indexing material from journals relevant to one or more professions or to a subject area. (Research tip 2.1 lists some of the databases that collate nursing and midwifery journal articles.) It is important to note that even within a specific discipline, not all relevant journals are indexed in any one database. A thorough search for available evidence includes searching a number of databases to ensure nothing has been missed. Hospital and university libraries also usually have a searchable catalogue that contains all of the material that they hold or subscribe to. Searching the catalogue can prove useful for finding assignment information, but catalogues also have their drawbacks, the main one being that they are only available to employees or students of the particular institution, and therefore the search cannot be replicated by anyone outside. This is important if you need to show exactly how you obtained the material.

Let us now turn to our case study and consider the steps involved in searching a database. Laura has decided to use MEDLINE to search for evidence on barriers to nurses washing their hands. Note that at this stage Laura's topic is expressed as a phrase, rather than as a question. If you do not know very much about a topic and what sort of research has been done on it, this is a good way to start. If Laura found that there was a great deal of literature on her topic, she could then refine it; for instance, she might decide to concentrate on strategies to overcome barriers, or, if there was a lot of literature, to look at whether one specific strategy was effective. For now, we will stick with the broader topic.

If Laura searched using the phrase **barriers to nurses washing their hands**, the database would attempt to find that exact phrase. While it may

RESEARCH TIP 2.1 Useful databases for finding nursing and midwifery research articles

Cochrane Library	Systematic reviews and meta-analyses
CINAHL	Cumulative Index to Nursing and Allied Health Literature
DOAJ	Directory of Open Access Journals
EMBASE	Biomedical literature
Joanna Briggs Institute	Best-practice information and systematic reviews
MEDLINE	Medical, nursing and allied health literature (closely related to PubMed)
MIDIRS	Maternity and infant care
Proquest	Nursing and allied health database
PsycINFO	Psychology and mental health
PubMed	Medical and allied health literature

have been used in some articles, it is almost certain that variations on the wording would also have been used, and these articles would not be found. The first step, then, is to identify the key concepts in the topic—these are called *search terms*. In Laura's case, the search terms are *handwashing*, *barriers* and *nurses*.

There are a number of ways to perform a search using the identified search terms. One way is to enter these terms directly into the database's search function—this is called *keyword searching*. In this strategy the database will search for the term exactly as it is entered. However, these exact terms may not have been used in all relevant articles, so it is important to think of potential synonyms. For instance, rather than *barriers*, some authors may have used the term *obstacles*.

To include all of the relevant concepts in the search, the keywords have to be combined. This can be done in two ways: entering keywords in a single search, or searching for each term individually and then combining the results. In both strategies, the combination is performed using **Boolean operators**—these are *AND*, *OR* and *NOT*. Each works in a different way. Using *AND* will return results that contain *all* of the included terms. This is used to combine the major concepts—for instance, **handwashing AND barriers AND nurses**. Using *OR* will return results that include at least one of the terms; it is mainly used to combine synonyms—in this example, **barriers OR obstacles**. The Boolean operator *NOT* will return results that include the first term but exclude the second; it can be useful to exclude a particular subset of articles that are not wanted. For example, Laura may want to exclude articles relating to surgical scrubbing; in this case, she might use the search **handwashing NOT surgical scrubbing**.

Boolean operator
a term used to combine keywords or search results in specific ways; terms available are *AND*, *OR* and *NOT*

Another issue to be aware of is that certain words can be spelt in different ways, while others can be used in different grammatical forms. Keyword searching will identify only articles that use the same spelling or form that you have used. Spelling usually varies by a single letter—for instance, *oesophagus* in the United Kingdom and Australia is spelt *esophagus* in the United States, and *paediatric* as *pediatric*. Both spellings can be included in a search (for example, **oesophagus OR esophagus**). However,

wildcard
a symbol used in place of a single letter to enable database searching for all variations of spelling

most databases have a **wildcard** option that allows the searcher to insert a character in the place of a letter that may or may not be present; the specific character varies between databases but in MEDLINE is a question mark. The keyword in this example would be entered as *?esophagus*. Variations can also occur in forms of words: in Laura's example, the concept of *nurses* may have been expressed by different authors as *nurse* or *nursing*. Rather than including every variation on the term in her search, Laura can use a **truncator** symbol to do this for her: the terms are reduced to their common letters—in this case, *nurs*—and the truncator symbol is placed after them. In MEDLINE, the truncator symbol is an asterisk. In this example, the keyword will be entered as *nurs**. Note that truncation can also return unwanted results. For example, *nurs* is also the beginning of the word *nursery*. Including this term might find articles relating to childcare centres or kindergartens. Laura could exclude these by using the Boolean operator *NOT*: *nurs* NOT nursery*.

truncator
a symbol used at the end of part of a word in a database search to enable searching for all words that begin with the same letters

---

ACTIVITY 2.1 Searching a database

1   On your institution's library website, go to a database of your choice.
2   Read the information provided about the database to determine what the wildcard and truncator characters are in that database.
3   Using the keywords identified in the text above, carry out a search to find articles relating to barriers to nurses washing their hands.

Question for consideration

• Which parts of the search did you find difficult? Review these areas with your lecturer or a colleague.

As we have seen, when using keywords to perform a search, it is important to identify all the synonyms that may have been used in the literature. The drawback to this method is that if you miss some synonyms, you will not find literature that you may need. A way around this is to locate your search term within an established thesaurus of terms, or subject headings. These differ somewhat between databases. One thesaurus that is used by several databases, including MEDLINE, was developed and maintained by the US National Library of Medicine, and is called **Medical Subject Headings** (MeSH). Mapping, or linking, terms to subject headings ensures that all related terms are searched for.

Medical Subject Headings
a thesaurus of terms maintained by the US National Library of Medicine; also known as MeSH

In MEDLINE, Laura types *handwashing* into the search bar and clicks on the box 'Map term to Subject Heading'. This takes Laura to a screen indicating that her term mapped to the MeSH term *hand disinfection*. At this point she has a number of options. We will concentrate on two: a link labelled 'Continue' and a link from the MeSH term itself.

When Laura clicks on the box labelled 'Continue', she can see all of the subheadings that have been used to index articles under this subject heading. If one or more of these were relevant to her topic, she could narrow her search at this point by ticking the relevant boxes. In this case, however, none is appropriate to her chosen topic, so she returns to the previous screen. By clicking on the subject heading itself she can see what is called the *tree*—the more specific and more general terms associated with the term. This tells her that the term above it—the more general term—in the tree is *hand hygiene*. She can also see how many articles are associated with each term. For each term, she can click on the information icon to see the *Scope* note—the definition of each term, how it has been indexed previously, related terms and all of the terms that are included under this heading:

MeSH heading: **hand disinfection**
Scope: The act of cleansing the hands with water or other liquid, with or without the inclusion of soap or other detergent, for the purpose of destroying infectious microorganisms. Used for:

- disinfection, hand
- sanitisation, hand
- hand disinfection
- scrubbing, surgical
- hand sanitisation
- surgical scrubbing
- hand washing
- washing, hand
- hand washings
- washings, hand
- handwashing.

MeSH heading: **hand hygiene**
Scope: Practices involved in preventing the transmission
of diseases by hand. Used for:

- hand hygiene
- hygiene, hand. (Ovid Technologies 2018)

Laura can now decide which of the terms she wants to use, or she can select both. To include both terms in her search, she will need to combine them using the Boolean operator *OR*. She also has the option of ticking boxes either to *explode* the search (to include the term and any more specific terms) or to *focus* it (limit the search to articles in which the term is the major focus). Laura elects to choose both *hand hygiene* and *hand disinfection* and to tick the 'Focus' boxes for each. This operation elicits more than 3500 articles—more than twice as many as were discovered by searching for the keyword *handwashing*.

MeSH headings are usually only useful for the main concept in a search, but it is worth trying the other terms to see if there is a suitable heading. *Barriers*, for instance, maps to a range of headings that have nothing to do with Laura's topic. *Nurses* is a MeSH term but retrieves only 5 per cent of the articles identified by the keyword search for *nurs**. Unless the final search result elicits too many articles to reasonably examine, it is usually best to use a search strategy that will give the most results.

Once Laura has combined the searches on the individual terms (using the operator *AND*), she can narrow the results even further by using the 'Limits' function. One limit used frequently is the publication year. Whether to use this and which years to choose depend on the purpose of the search. If you want to know the most recent findings on a topic, restricting the search to the last five or ten years is a useful rule of thumb. However, if you want to know whether *any* research on your topic has been undertaken, you may need to go back further. For example, the link between lack of hand hygiene by healthcare workers and infections among patients is well established, and you would be unlikely to find recent research on that exact topic. (You might, however, find research on the comparative effectiveness of different types of hand hygiene.) There may be a specific time point at which practices changed (for example, the introduction of new laws or guidelines) that would influence the literature on a topic, so it would make sense to search for articles published only after that date. In Laura's case, she will need to retrieve articles only from the last five years, to comply with her assignment instructions. Another available option is to limit the search to articles written in English; this can be useful if the searcher can read no other languages and does not have translation resources. If relevant to the topic, other limits that can be applied include people's ages, types of articles and subsets of journals or subjects. Another option is 'Full text available'; this restricts the search to those articles to which the database has a full text link. This is not the same as a library's full text availability, which is any journal to which the institution subscribes. It is best, therefore, *not* to use this limit in your search, even when finding information for assignments.

TABLE 2.2 Results of searches conducted in MEDLINE concerning barriers to handwashing in nurses

Search number	Searches	Results
1	barriers to nurses washing their hands	0
2	hand hygiene OR hand disinfection [MeSH terms, focused]	3679
3	handwashing [keyword]	1631
4	barriers OR obstacles [keyword]	129486
5	nurs* [keyword, truncated]	644147
6	nurses [MeSH term]	35852
7	2 AND 4 AND 5	33
8	limit 7 to English language and year=2013-current	14
9	limit 8 to full text	4

Source: Adapted from Ovid Technologies 2018

All of the concepts we have discussed in this section are illustrated in Table 2.2, which shows the results of the various searches and the effects of applying limits. As we saw above, applying the full text limit excludes a significant number of articles that Laura could use in her assignment. The best search strategy in this case has given her fourteen articles to examine further. Note that no search strategy, however carefully designed, is foolproof, and there will likely be a number of retrieved citations that are not relevant to your specific topic. There is no way to avoid the final step, which is to read the titles and abstracts of the retrieved articles, to determine which ones will meet your needs.

ACTIVITY 2.2 Constructing a strategy to search the literature

Choose any topic of interest to you and consider how you will go about finding research evidence on that topic.

Questions for consideration
- Which databases are likely to include articles relevant to your topic?
- Are there any MeSH terms relevant to your topic?
- What keywords could you use? Could these be spelt in different ways? What synonyms might have been used for these terms?
- How will you combine these terms in a search?

How do I judge evidence?

In Chapter 1 we introduced you to the concept of hierarchies of evidence. This concept is underpinned by the fact that research evidence can be generated using several approaches, or study designs, and these do not all provide the same weight of evidence. Put simply, some designs are better suited to answering certain types of questions than others. Hierarchies of evidence were first developed to consider questions of effectiveness of various practices in producing a particular outcome, and they enable us to judge how confident we can be that the results of a study are 'real', or valid. For example, in Research example 1.4 in the previous chapter, we looked at a systematic review that asked how effective the World Health Organization's hand hygiene campaign had been in improving hand hygiene compliance in healthcare workers. The evidence hierarchy in this example helps us to judge whether the reported increase in compliance was due to the campaign or to some other factor. Some study designs include elements that enable us to have more confidence in the findings; hence, some designs are ranked higher than others. We will discuss these designs, and their various elements, in detail in subsequent chapters. A number of organisations have published evidence hierarchies; in Australia, we usually use the one produced by the National Health and Medical Research Council (see Chapter 1) or the more detailed and more recent one published by the Joanna Briggs Institute (2014). In these hierarchies the various types of studies (described in Chapter 4) are assigned to a numbered level, which makes it easy to describe the quality of evidence when preparing literature reviews (see Chapter 9) and clinical practice guidelines (see Chapter 8). The levels of evidence relevant to studies of practice effectiveness are reproduced in Table 2.3.

Evidence-based health care is not simply about practice effectiveness, however; healthcare professionals have other questions, and research approaches designed to answer those questions can also provide evidence for practice. Other evidence hierarchies address those approaches. In nursing and midwifery, we are often interested in people's experiences, perceptions or behaviours, using qualitative approaches (see Chapter 5) to answer these questions. These concerns are categorised by the Joanna Briggs Institute (2014) as questions of 'meaningfulness'. The JBI has produced an evidence hierarchy for these types of studies:

1   Qualitative or mixed methods systematic review
2   Qualitative or mixed methods synthesis
3   Single qualitative study
4   Systematic review of expert opinion
5   Expert opinion. (Joanna Briggs Institute 2014)

The level of evidence tells us about the quality of the available evidence—how credible it is. However, when deciding whether or not to incorporate

TABLE 2.3 Joanna Briggs Institute's levels of evidence for studies of effectiveness, highest to lowest

Level 1   Experimental designs
        Level 1.a   Systematic review of randomised controlled trials (RCTs)
        Level 1.b   Systematic review of RCTs and other study designs
        Level 1.c   RCT
        Level 1.d   Pseudo-RCTs

Level 2   Quasi-experimental designs
        Level 2.a   Systematic review of quasi-experimental studies
        Level 2.b   Systematic review of quasi-experimental and other lower study designs
        Level 2.c   Quasi-experimental prospectively controlled study
        Level 2.d   Pre-test–post-test or historic/retrospective control group study

Level 3   Observational: analytic designs
        Level 3.a   Systematic review of comparable cohort studies
        Level 3.b   Systematic review of comparable cohort and other lower study designs
        Level 3.c   Cohort study with control group
        Level 3.d   Case-controlled study
        Level 3.e   Observational study without a control group

Level 4   Observational: descriptive studies
        Level 4.a   Systematic review of descriptive studies
        Level 4.b   Cross-sectional study
        Level 4.c   Case series
        Level 4.d   Case study

Level 5   Expert opinion and bench research
        Level 5.a   Systematic review of expert opinion
        Level 5.b   Expert consensus
        Level 5.c   Bench research/single expert opinion

Source: Joanna Briggs Institute 2014

specific evidence into our practice, a number of other factors have to be taken into consideration. This topic is explored in more detail in Chapter 8, in the discussion of clinical practice guidelines. Briefly, recommendations for the use of evidence in practice are graded as strong or weak and take into account the feasibility and appropriateness of a practice, as well as its meaningfulness and effectiveness (Joanna Briggs Institute 2014).

ACTIVITY 2.3 Levels of evidence

1 Using the search strategy you developed in Activity 2.2, choose any two of the retrieved research reports.
2 Examine how the authors describe the type of research (which may be called *design*, *method* or *methodology* depending on the approach and the journal's style).
3 Try to identify the level of evidence that would be ascribed to the research.

Questions for consideration

- Was it easy or difficult to identify the level of evidence? Why was that?
- If it was difficult, what additional information could the authors have provided to assist in making this identification?

RESEARCH EXAMPLE 2.1 Do nurses source research evidence?

Nurses have a professional responsibility to use evidence in their practice; this is especially the case for nurses in clinical leadership roles. Malik et al. (2015) surveyed 135 nurse educators, clinical coaches and nurse specialists to explore their perceptions of and skills in evidence-based practice. One question concerned sources of the knowledge they used in their practice. They found that the most commonly used sources of knowledge were organisational policies and protocols, and personal experience. Research journals ranked second lowest as a source of information. Overall, participants rated their skills in finding research evidence as low.

G. Malik, L. McKenna & V. Plummer, 2015, 'Perceived knowledge, skills, attitude and contextual factors affecting evidence-based practice among nurse educators, clinical coaches and nurse specialists', *International Journal of Nursing Practice*, vol. 21, pp. 46–57, doi: 10.1111/ijn.12366.

Questions for consideration

- What do you consider to be the implications of these findings for nursing practice?
- What strategies could be put in place to increase nurses' skills in finding and using research evidence?

CHAPTER SUMMARY

Locating high-quality evidence is a vital first step in evidence-based practice. This chapter has examined potential sources of research evidence and considered the relative credibility of each. Strategies to locate research evidence have been described. The need to consider the quality and strength of evidence when making decisions about its use in practice has been considered.

CHAPTER REVIEW QUESTIONS

- What are the best sources for nursing and midwifery research evidence?
- Why are some sources considered better than others?
- What steps would you undertake in finding research evidence on a specific topic?
- What are Boolean operators? What functions do they perform?
- What do hierarchies of evidence tell us?

QUESTIONS FOR DISCUSSION

- Why is it important for nurses and midwives to undertake effective literature searches?
- Why is it important to understand evidence quality? How does this impact on clinical practice?

QUESTIONS FOR PERSONAL REFLECTION

- What have you learnt about finding and evaluating research evidence while working through this chapter?
- How can you incorporate this knowledge into your practice?

USEFUL WEB RESOURCES

Joanna Briggs Institute <http://joannabriggs.org>
National Health and Medical Research Council on research <www.nhmrc.gov.au/research>
US National Library of Medicine's Medical Subject Headings <www.nlm.nih.gov/mesh/>

REFERENCES AND FURTHER READING

Aromataris, E. & Riitano, D., 2014, 'Constructing a search strategy and search for evidence: A guide to the literature search for a systematic review', *American Journal of Nursing*, vol. 114, no. 5, pp. 49–56.

Baillie, L., 2015, 'Disseminating research', *Nurse Researcher*, vol. 22, no. 6, pp. 6–7.

Beyea, S., 2000, 'Finding internet resources to support evidence-based practice', *AORN Journal*, vol. 72, no. 3, pp. 514–515.

Childs, G.M., 2009, 'Finding evidence-based practice information', *Physical & Occupational Therapy in Pediatrics*, vol. 29, no. 4, pp. 337–344.

Considine, J., Shaban, R.Z., Fry, M. & Curtis, K., 2017, 'Evidence based emergency nursing: Designing a research question and searching the literature', *International Emergency Nursing*, vol. 32, pp. 78–82.

Facchiano, L. & Hoffman Snyder, C., 2012, 'Evidence-based practice for the busy nurse practitioner', part 2: 'Searching for the best evidence to clinical inquiries', *Journal of the American Academy of Nurse Practitioners*, vol. 24, pp. 640–648.

Joanna Briggs Institute, 2014, *Levels of Evidence*, <http://joannabriggs.org/jbi-approach.html#tabbed-nav=Levels-of-Evidence>.

Malik, G., McKenna, L. & Plummer, V., 2015, 'Perceived knowledge, skills, attitude and contextual factors affecting evidence-based practice among nurse educators, clinical coaches and nurse specialists', *International Journal of Nursing Practice*, vol. 21, pp. 46–57, doi: 10.1111/ijn.12366.

National Health and Medical Research Council *see* NHMRC

NHMRC, 2009, *NHMRC Levels of Evidence and Grades for Recommendations for Developers of Guidelines*, <www.nhmrc.gov.au/_files_nhmrc/file/guidelines/developers/nhmrc_levels_grades_evidence_120423.pdf>.

Ovid Technologies, 2018, MEDLINE, database, US National Library of Medicine (details at <www.ovid.com/site/catalog/databases/901.jsp>).

Power, A. & Siddall, G., 2015, 'Ensuring practice is based on the best evidence: Masterclass on literature searching', *British Journal of Midwifery*, vol. 23, no. 5, pp. 356–358.

Raines, D.A., 2013, 'Finding the evidence', *Neonatal Network*, vol. 32, no. 3, pp. 203–205.

Salmond, S.W., 2014, 'Finding the evidence to support evidence-based practice', *Orthopaedic Nursing*, vol. 32, no. 1, pp. 16–22.

Stillwell, S.B., Fineout-Overholt, E., Melnyk, B.M. & Williamson, K.M., 2010, 'Searching for the evidence: Strategies to help you conduct a successful search', *American Journal of Nursing*, vol. 110, no. 5, pp. 41–47.

Wyer, P.C., Allen, T.Y. & Corrall, C.J., 2004, 'Finding evidence when you need it', *Evidence-Based Cardiovascular Medicine* vol. 8, pp. 2–7.

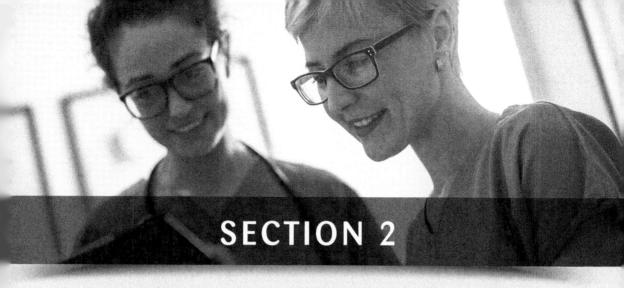

SECTION 2

HOW CAN I MAKE SENSE OF RESEARCH EVIDENCE?

Section 1 introduced the reader to evidence-based practice in nursing and midwifery along with the need for nurses and midwives to understand research in order to inform practice. Trying to understand research papers can be daunting at first. They often use language and concepts that are new and appear complex. This section is focused on breaking down some of that complexity and providing the reader with a base on which to build research knowledge.

Chapter 3 introduces the research process. In doing so, it steps through each of the stages in conducting a research study, as well as some of the considerations needed. It introduces the concepts of quantitative and qualitative research, which are then built upon further in Chapters 4 and 5, employing a focus on person-centred care to illustrate their characteristics.

Chapter 4 introduces quantitative approaches to research, involving numerical, or statistical, analysis. The chapter presents basic statistical concepts commonly employed in nursing and midwifery research.

Chapter 5 introduces qualitative approaches to research, highlighting that these are particularly common in nursing and midwifery. It also discusses common approaches to data collection and data analysis, as well as ensuring research quality.

CHAPTER 3

Understanding how research is done

LEARNING OBJECTIVES

After working through this chapter, you should be able to:

- describe the steps in the research process
- outline the key differences between qualitative and quantitative approaches
- define a *population* and a *sample*
- identify potential sources of research data
- outline formal and informal processes for gaining approval to undertake research
- outline strategies for disseminating research findings
- identify challenges that nurses and midwives might experience in collecting research data.

KEY TERMS AND CONCEPTS

Analysis, approval, data collection, population, qualitative, quantitative, research process, research proposal, research question, sample

CASE STUDY OVERVIEW

A large hospital has a strong philosophy that health care should be person centred. At a meeting of senior nurses, there is a discussion around whether and how this translates into nursing practice. Nurse unit managers consider their own wards and departments and identify a number of issues and concerns. Some are uncertain about the extent to which person-centred care is being delivered and think this needs to be determined before proceeding with any further work. Others are certain that there are deficiencies in the delivery of person-centred care in their departments. Some of these think they should examine the reasons behind this, and others would like to look at ways of improving person-centred care.

CHAPTER INTRODUCTION

Whether nurses and midwives want to undertake their own research or use existing evidence in their practice, an understanding of how research is actually carried out is fundamental to effective care. Every research study consists of a number of steps, which are known collectively as the research process. (This was described briefly in Chapter 1.) The steps may not always be followed in exactly the same order, and the process may or may not be linear—sometimes steps can be revisited several times—but in general terms, the process is universal. This chapter describes in more detail the steps involved in planning and undertaking research. It introduces several concepts that will be explored in more depth in subsequent chapters.

Getting started: Where do research questions come from?

Ideas for research can come from anywhere, but essentially they arise from a questioning attitude or from taking a critical approach to what we do. Ideally, we would constantly be asking questions about our practice—Why do we do something this way? Could we do it better?—but in the bustle of everyday life it is very easy to just accept things the way they are. Questioning can be facilitated in a number of ways: reading journal articles, going to conferences, talking to colleagues (particularly those in other departments or hospitals), listening to those for whom we care or simply reflecting regularly on our work.

Research begins with a broad topic of interest. In this chapter's case study, **person-centred care** is the broad topic. From this, researchers identify an issue or problem that they wish to address. In the case study, these problems are:

- uncertainty about whether person-centred care is delivered
- wanting to understand why person-centred care is not being delivered consistently
- wanting to improve the delivery of person-centred care.

person-centred care
care that is focused on the person and in which the person is given autonomy to make decisions about their care

Practice does not have to be perceived as a problem in order for us to investigate it. Rather than asking why something does not work, we might ask why it does! For instance, staff in some wards might decide that they practise person-centred care very well indeed; they and other staff would be interested in what enabled staff in that ward to practise person-centred care when staff in other wards did not. In practical terms, though, it is usually much harder to question something that is working well than something that has obvious problems.

The issues or problems listed above are still quite broad and are not specific enough to guide a research study. They need to be refined further to generate focused questions that can be answered through research. Within any broad topic, and often within issues or problems, there are several research questions that can be asked. Some examples of possible research questions arising from the issues listed above are:

- To what extent is person-centred care being practised throughout the hospital?
- What are the factors that facilitate or prevent the practice of person-centred care?
- What are nurses' perceptions and understandings of person-centred care?
- What are patients' perspectives of the practice of person-centred care?
- Can a nursing education program improve the practice of person-centred care?

When reading research reports, you will probably find that questions such as the ones listed above are not actually included. More commonly, the **research aim** is expressed

research aim
what a researcher is seeking to achieve by doing a study

as a statement. However, it is important to realise that the aim of any research study is to find the answer to a question, whether expressed as such or not—it is, effectively, to generate new knowledge. The aim of a study is not to change practice or improve patient outcomes; this is the significance of a study, or what you hope to achieve with the findings. It is helpful, therefore, to express an aim in the form of a question rather than a statement, because it focuses on the desired answer.

Moving from a problem to a **research question** requires some understanding of the topic and of what research has already been undertaken. Therefore, a literature review is usually undertaken at this stage. One reason for doing this is to identify gaps in current knowledge. It may be that there is already sufficient research evidence on a particular topic and the identified problem can best be addressed by implementing this evidence. It is unethical to conduct research unnecessarily—a topic we will explore further in Chapter 7. If more research is found to be justified, the literature review can be helpful in planning the study. Replicating another researcher's design makes it easier to compare findings across studies. The literature review can further help to refine the question by identifying existing measurement tools (to measure person-centred care, in this example) or interventions (like an education program) that have previously been tested.

research question
the question that a research study is designed to answer

RESEARCH EXAMPLE 3.1 Why do a literature review?

There is a great deal of literature, in nursing and other health professions, on the topic of person-centred care. Sharma et al. (2015, p. 108) undertook an overview of reviews that addressed the following questions:

1   What is person-centred care?
2   What nursing or healthcare provider behaviours demonstrate a person-centred approach during the delivery of care to a person?
3   What are the evidence-based models of care delivery, which demonstrate effective outcomes that support person-centred care?

4   What components of person-centred care should be taught in basic curricula or ongoing professional education programs?

5   What organisational or system structures support successful implementation of person-centred care?

The researchers identified 46 reviews that met their criteria. They found that the concept of person-centred care was poorly defined, but they were able to identify components that were common across studies, healthcare-provider behaviours commonly associated with person-centred care and the organisational supports required for its practice.

T. Sharma, M. Bamford & D. Dodman, 2015, 'Person-centred care: An overview of reviews', *Contemporary Nurse*, vol. 51, nos 2–3, pp. 107–120.

Questions for consideration

- How might this paper assist staff in our case study to refine their research question?
- How else might it be useful to someone planning research on this topic?

Selecting an approach

There are two main broad approaches to undertaking research, known as *quantitative* and *qualitative*, which will be discussed in depth in the next two chapters. Here, we provide a brief overview, highlighting differences between the two approaches; these are summarised in Table 3.1.

It is important to understand that all research approaches are underpinned by a particular view of the world (known as a **paradigm**) that includes assumptions about the nature of reality, about what it means to be a person and about how knowledge can and should be generated. You will often see the word **methodology** used to encompass how these beliefs and assumptions shape the way research is undertaken (Grant & Giddings 2002). The two research approaches are useful for answering different kinds of questions; therefore, the question will

paradigm
a particular viewpoint of the world

methodology
the philosophical beliefs or assumptions that influence a study's design

TABLE 3.1 Differences between quantitative and qualitative research approaches

Attribute	Quantitative	Qualitative
View	Objective	Subjective
Perspective	One truth or answer	Multiple truths
Focus	What, how much	How, why
Design	Usually fixed	Usually evolving
Data types	Numbers, information	Words, text, pictures
Data analysis	Statistical	Content, thematic

tend to determine which approach is chosen. However, the researcher's own philosophical beliefs will also influence the choice: they are more likely to be interested in asking questions that are best answered by the approach that aligns most closely with their beliefs.

Quantitative research

Quantitative research can be thought of as relating to numbers. It is primarily concerned with *measuring* concepts of interest and often with comparing the measurements to test theories. Questions about the effectiveness of practices—Do they have the effect we want to see? Are they better than other practices? If so, by how much?—are addressed using a quantitative approach. Quantitative methods are based on the assumptions that there is one *truth*, or answer, to the questions posed and that researchers (and all of the methods used) must remain objective in order to discover the truth. All elements of the research design are determined before commencing, with little opportunity for change once the research is under way. Data for quantitative studies are collected or expressed numerically and analysed using statistical methods.

Qualitative research

Qualitative research can be thought of as relating to words and behaviours, with findings 'telling a story' to answer the research question. It is concerned with how people experience, perceive or understand the concept of interest or with why they behave in certain ways (Miller 2010). Qualitative approaches are based on the assumption that there are multiple *truths*—that people define their own reality, either as individuals or as part of a social group—and that no individual view is more or less true than another (Taylor & Francis 2013). In other words, everything we research using these approaches is inherently subjective. Qualitative research designs often evolve as the research progresses: the number of participants, data sources and exact kinds of data may change as new information emerges.

ACTIVITY 3.1 Questions suitable for quantitative and qualitative approaches

---

Read the list of possible research questions relating to the broad topic of person-centred care earlier in this chapter.

Questions for consideration

- Which questions would be best answered using a quantitative design? Why?
- Which would be appropriate for a qualitative design? Why?

Mixed methods research

A third research approach, **mixed methods**, usually involves combining quantitative and qualitative approaches. This approach is useful for answering the complex questions that often arise in clinical practice or for addressing a series of questions on the same topic to solve a practice problem (Cresswell & Plano-Clark 2018). For example, researchers might use a qualitative approach first (for instance, to understand why person-centred care is not practised in a specific ward)

mixed methods
a research approach involving mixing of more than one research method in one study, usually combining quantitative and qualitative approaches

and then a quantitative approach (to evaluate an intervention to improve practice). Researchers undertaking quantitative experimental studies (see Chapter 4) to see if new practices improve patient outcomes often include a qualitative component to understand patients' experiences of the new practice. Thus, mixed methods studies aim to produce more rounded findings that are better able to influence practice than either quantitative or qualitative approaches alone. A mixed methods approach is complex, requiring skills and knowledge beyond simply understanding each of the component approaches, and we will not be considering it in depth in this text.

RESEARCH EXAMPLE 3.2 Using mixed methods to study person-centred nursing care

---

Person-centred care of children—usually called *child- and family-centred care—* is believed to be fundamental in ensuring children's and their families' wellbeing. However, little is known of how it is practised outside Western countries. Alabdulaziz et al. (2017) wanted to understand whether and how nurses in Saudi Arabia practised family-centred care. They conducted a mixed methods study to answer this question. First, they surveyed nurses to find out which aspects of family-centred care they thought were important and which they actually practised (quantitative component). Then, they interviewed nurses and observed their interactions with families (qualitative component). The qualitative findings provided understandings of and explanations for the quantitative findings, thus providing a more complete answer to the research question.

H. Alabdulaziz, C. Moss & B. Copnell, 2017, 'Paediatric nurses' perceptions and practices of family-centred care in Saudi hospitals: A mixed methods study', *International Journal of Nursing Studies*, vol. 69, pp. 66–77.

Questions for consideration
- Why was a mixed methods approach useful for this study?
- What might be the limitations of this study if the researchers had only chosen one method?

ACTIVITY 3.2 Differences between quantitative and qualitative research

1 Search for two research articles on a topic of interest to you, one quantitative and one qualitative.
2 Carefully read both articles, taking particular note of the research question or aim, the methods and the presentation of the findings.

Questions for consideration

• What differences do you see in the ways the studies are reported?
• Was the approach used in each of the papers appropriate? Why?
• Could the questions have been answered another way?
• What do you consider to be the strengths of each study?
• Which of the articles did you find easier to read? Why?
• Which of the studies did you find easier to relate to? Why?

Writing the research proposal

As part of the research planning process, researchers usually write a proposal, which is a blueprint for their intended study. A proposal can be written solely for the research team, to ensure everyone has the same understanding of what will be involved. Often, though, it is intended for external use: to gain approval by an ethics committee or an institution, or to obtain funding. The exact format varies somewhat, depending on the purpose, but generally describes how the researchers will complete each of the steps in the research process (see below).

A good research proposal sets the scene for the proposed study. It justifies the need for the study, by exploring what is already known on the topic and identifying a gap in current knowledge that the proposed research will fill. It has a clearly expressed aim and contains detailed but concise descriptions of all procedures. The importance, or significance, of the research, both to the wider community and to specific stakeholders, must be clear. Ethical considerations are usually discussed. Proposals intended for external scrutiny, such as by funding bodies, must convince their readers that the study can be conducted: the researchers have sufficient knowledge of their topic and expertise in research to undertake the study; there is sufficient time to complete the study (a detailed time-frame is usually included); and there are sufficient resources to complete the study, or the requested funding is appropriate (this requires submission of a detailed budget). Research proposals are examined in more detail in Chapter 10.

Seeking approval

Before the study can begin, researchers have to obtain approval from a number of sources. The first priority is ensuring all the proposed procedures are ethical. All research involving humans must be reviewed by one or more ethics committees. Approval is also required from the institution in which the research is to be undertaken—that is, where the research participants are located—and usually from the institution where the researchers are located, if this is different. For instance, university staff or students undertaking research in a hospital would need approval from both the university and the hospital. We will look in detail at what constitutes ethical research, and the work of ethics committees, in Chapter 7.

Permission to undertake the study might also be required from other people or institutions. The head of a department where the research will be undertaken will probably need to allow access to the department, to ensure that normal work is not disrupted by the research. This approval process often forms part of the ethical review. If participants are not within a specific institution but sought through other channels (such as professional organisations, support groups, social networks and so on), those bodies will need to approve the study. For some specific types of research, notification of various bodies is required. For example, research involving drugs or devices that are either not registered in Australia or not approved for use in the way they will be used in the research must be reported to the Therapeutic Goods Administration, which will monitor the progress of the study. All randomised controlled trials (see Chapter 4) must be registered in a publicly accessible database before participants are enrolled (World Medical Association 2013). This is partly to ensure that the study and therefore its findings are genuine and partly to assist people who might benefit from participating in a trial to find studies that could be suitable for them. There are international trial registries, but many countries have their own. The Australian and New Zealand Clinical Trials Registry can be accessed at <www.anzctr.org.au>.

Formal approval and notification processes are not researchers' only considerations. Informal processes can also come into play if key people in the research setting can influence how, or indeed whether, the research is undertaken. These people are known as *gatekeepers*, and their cooperation is crucial in successfully conducting research. Gatekeepers may have a role in providing access to potential participants, perhaps notifying a member of the research team of suitable candidates or passing information to people who might be participants. Sometimes, particularly in larger studies, staff may be asked to comply with study procedures; for instance, clinicians may need to carry out a specific nursing or midwifery practice in a specific way. A number of factors can influence gatekeepers' cooperation. Research that is seen as burdensome or difficult for clinicians or the department as a whole, particularly if it impacts on workload, is less likely to elicit cooperation. Similarly, staff are less likely to comply with procedures they perceive to be harmful or potentially harmful to patients (whether or not their perceptions are accurate) or if they see the research as unimportant. Even when they wish to cooperate, however, busy clinicians can forget about research in the press of daily work. The attitude of researchers can have a considerable influence on gatekeepers. Requesting assistance and rewarding compliance are more likely to produce a favourable response than complaints and recriminations.

Selecting participants

Before making decisions about who will take part in the research, we first need to identify the target **population**—the people who will be the focus of the research question. A population is defined as a group of people with common characteristics to whom we want the results of our research to apply. Usually, this means the people we can access. In any of the possible

population
the entire group of people to whom researchers want to apply their findings

studies being undertaken in our case study, the population might be all nurses in the hospital. However, if we believe there are important differences between the practices of nurses in various departments, the population will be defined as nurses working in a department or ward where the study is taking place. If we want our population to be 'all nurses working in medical wards in public hospitals in Australia', we will need to include a number of such hospitals in the study to be able to apply our findings to this group.

Sometimes it is possible to study all of the population, particularly if it comprises a relatively small number of individuals. In the above example, for instance, it would (at least theoretically) be possible to involve all of the nurses in one ward or one hospital in a study. In other cases, research designs have been developed that allow researchers to study very large populations, such as all women giving birth in Australia. More often, though, it is not practical to include the entire population, so researchers must choose a subset to take part in the research. The subset is called a **sample**, and the act of selecting it is known as **sampling**. There are several ways of selecting a study sample; these vary between qualitative and quantitative approaches and even within each approach. We will discuss these in detail in the following chapters.

sample
the subset of a population selected to take part in the research

sampling
the process of selecting research participants

The sampling method is not the only decision researchers have to make with respect to their participants. They must also decide where they will recruit people (that is, what the study setting will be) and how many participants they need (the sample size). How this decision is made depends mainly on the research design. Researchers need to establish what characteristics they want the participants to have and whether there are characteristics that they do not want. These requirements are called **inclusion** and **exclusion criteria**. They also have to decide on a recruitment strategy—how they will let potential participants know about the study and, in turn, how people will let the researchers know they want to take part. Sometimes, researchers approach potential participants directly, in

inclusion criteria
characteristics that a potential participant or a study must possess to be included in research or a literature review

exclusion criteria
characteristics that exclude a participant from a study or a study from a review

person; this is the commonest method when conducting clinical research with patients, for instance. In some situations, it may not be possible or desirable for the researchers to approach individuals directly. They may instead advertise the study by means of flyers in the settings where they want to recruit, in newspapers, by email sent via a contact (for example, nurse unit managers may be asked to send an email to all their staff, or a professional organisation to its members) or on social media platforms, such as Facebook and Twitter. In all strategies, researchers must have plans for providing people with information about the study and obtaining their consent to take part (we will discuss this further in Chapter 7), and for how those who agree will either contact the researchers or provide their data.

ACTIVITY 3.3 Research considerations

A great deal of preparation goes into a research study. Summarise in a series of bullet points what you see to be the key considerations in planning a study.

Collecting data

The term **data** refers to any information collected to answer the research question. Data can be classified as inherently *quantitative* (that is, the information exists in a numerical format: a person's age, weight, body temperature and so on) or as *qualitative*, or non-numerical (a person's gender, hair colour, favourite food, opinion about a particular issue and so on). In practice, this distinction is only partially useful, however.

data
information collected to answer a research question

data collection
the process of collecting data to answer a research question

Data can be collected in almost any format and from almost anywhere. Common sources are:

- **Directly from people themselves** Data can be collected by measuring physical attributes, either immediately (height and weight, blood pressure, temperature, etc.) or at a later time (for instance, collecting blood or urine to measure substances such as cholesterol or glucose). We can observe people in specific situations. We can ask questions of people, either in person or through another medium (such as a written or electronic survey).

- **Directly from the environment** We can measure attributes such as room temperature, noise levels, light levels and available space.

- **Existing data about individuals** This can be a very convenient way of obtaining data as it is usually less time consuming than sourcing it directly, although there are some disadvantages. Medical records are one such data source. Others are patient databases, which can exist at department, hospital/health service, state or even national level. Another example is patient registries, where details are recorded of patients with specific medical conditions (such as various cancers) or requiring specific types of care (such as intensive care admission).

- **Existing data about society or the context of a research project** This category can include policy documents, official records (such as incident reports in hospitals, birth and death records), published texts (books, newspapers, journal articles, etc.), and other media (film, television, etc.).

As well as deciding from where data will be collected, researchers must decide what data to collect. The data must enable the research question to be answered. This may sound simple (even obvious) but in reality can be complex and quite difficult. If the data are being collected by asking people questions, for instance, researchers must decide what questions to ask to get the information they want. Questions can be misunderstood by participants or just not specific enough to elicit the information. Even something as apparently straightforward as body temperature becomes more complicated when you consider that there are several sites on the body where temperature can be taken and several instruments that can be used to measure it, all of which might give slightly different readings. If we want to compare temperature across patients or across time periods, we need to take their temperature at the same site and using the same device every time. We also have to consider how many people will be collecting data. If more than one, it is important to ensure that everyone is collecting the data in the same way.

Other information must also be collected. Some demographic or clinical information will be needed to allow descriptions of the participants and enable the researchers (and those reading the research findings) to judge whether the sample is typical of the population or of a population in other settings. There is no standard list of items that should be included in demographic data. Rather, their relevance to the research question needs to be considered. Age might be important, for instance, when researching patients, as disease processes are likely to vary in different age groups. But if we are researching nurses' attitudes towards person-centred care, we might be less interested in their ages than in how long they have been practising as nurses. For research on patients, clinical data should be collected if it might influence the research outcome or help readers determine whether they should implement the findings. Finally, if the research involves the evaluation of an intervention, such as a new practice (see Chapter 4), the details of the intervention should be recorded to ensure that it is carried out in an identical way for all participants.

The format in which data will be collected also needs to be decided. A survey, for instance, could be paper based or electronic. If data collection is by **observation**, the situation might be filmed, or the observers may make notes about what they are seeing. Interviews with participants may be audio- or video-recorded, or the interviewer may write down the participants' responses. When physiological or clinical data are collected, they are usually recorded on a data collection form, which again may be in paper or electronic format.

observation
a data collection method where participants are observed in a specific context

---

ACTIVITY 3.4 Collecting research data

Data can be collected in many forms. Consider the possible challenges for nursing and midwifery researchers in collecting research data and suggest how these challenges might be managed.

Analysing data

Data analysis means making sense of the data that have been collected, in order to answer the research question. There are several ways in which this can be done, and they differ significantly between quantitative and qualitative approaches. In quantitative studies, statistical analysis is performed, and the results are presented in a numerical format. Often, tables and figures (such as graphs) are used to display the results. In qualitative studies, analysis is focused on finding patterns (themes or categories) in the data, and the findings are usually presented in narrative form. We will discuss specific methods of analysis in detail in the following two chapters.

Interpreting findings

This stage of the research process is undertaken to help consumers of research put the findings into context. You will see this stage in research reports under the heading 'Discussion'. The researchers consider how the findings of their particular study fit with what is already known on the topic: the findings may add further weight to a body of evidence, or they may challenge existing knowledge. Explanations should be suggested for new or unexpected findings; for example, the research may have been carried out in a different setting from that of previous studies or with people displaying different characteristics. The implications for practice (or policy or education, depending on the topic) should be discussed. Limitations of the study—factors that might restrict the application of the study's findings—should be identified. The researchers should also discuss what is still not known about the topic and suggest avenues for further research; there is a saying that good research asks more questions than it answers.

Communicating findings

The final stage of the research process is one that novice researchers often neglect to consider at the outset but is arguably the most important. If research findings are not communicated to others, the research might as well not have been done. It can be argued that failing to communicate findings is unethical, as people have taken part in research on the understanding that something useful will come of it. There are three groups of people to whom the findings should be communicated: participants, stakeholder groups and the wider scientific (and possibly lay) community. The communication of research findings is commonly referred to as **dissemination**.

dissemination
communication of research findings, for example, through publication or presentation

It is generally expected that people who have given up their time (at least) to take part in research should be given the opportunity to learn about its outcomes. Researchers are usually required, during preparation for the research, to formulate a plan for how they will communicate their findings. Normally, participants are told at the time of recruitment when the results are expected to be available and how to obtain them. If researchers have direct contact with the participants, they can offer to send them a summary of the findings. If there is no direct contact (in the case of an anonymous survey, for instance), the findings may be made available through a mutual contact.

Beyond the participants, a number of groups may have a specific interest in the study findings. Organisations that provide funding for research usually require a summary of the results. Approval bodies, such as ethics committees, often ask for a final report, which, while having a different focus, sometimes includes the study's findings. If research is undertaken in a specific organisation or environment, staff in the organisation will have a particular interest in the findings, as they are directly relevant to them. Staff will be specifically interested in the implications for their practice, especially if change is indicated.

For research to be relevant beyond the immediate setting, however, the findings have to be dispersed widely. This means they must be published in an academic journal, so that they can be read by both users of research and other researchers. This method of dissemination potentially reaches the biggest audience. Researchers can promote their work through a number of avenues to encourage others to read it, including social media platforms, blogs and membership of social networking sites like LinkedIn and ResearchGate. News media can also be used to draw attention to important research findings. Another useful way of disseminating findings to the scientific community is by presenting at conferences. This gives researchers direct contact with potential users of their research and with other researchers, allowing them to answer questions and discuss their work in detail. The disadvantage of this dissemination method is that a relatively small number of people are exposed to the research presented, compared with the potential audience of a journal article. Conference presentation should complement publication, not replace it.

ACTIVITY 3.5 Disseminating research findings through social media

Social media is a key mechanism by which scholars disseminate their research findings. There are a number of available social media platforms with which researchers should be familiar.

1 Go to one or more of the following websites:
   • ResearchGate
   • LinkedIn
   • Academic.edu
   • Google Scholar.
2 At each website, look for some researchers you may know in your discipline (for example, authors of articles you have read, your lecturers, people in clinical settings with whom you have worked). Note the types of information available on each site.

CHAPTER SUMMARY

Understanding how research is carried out is important for nurses and midwives, whether they want to do their own research or read research reports as the basis for decisions about their practice. In this chapter, we have explored the steps, or research process, involved in any research study. The first vital step is to generate an answerable research question located within what is already known on the topic through undertaking a literature review. There are two main approaches to research—quantitative and qualitative—and we have examined the differences between them. A third approach, mixed methods, was described briefly. The approach selected will guide subsequent steps, including selecting participants, collecting data and analysing data. Finally, it is vital to communicate research findings to others.

CHAPTER REVIEW QUESTIONS

- What are the key differences between quantitative and qualitative approaches to research?
- What are the key decisions researchers must make in relation to how they carry out research?
- From what sources can data be collected?
- What strategies can researchers use to communicate their findings?

QUESTIONS FOR DISCUSSION

- How can nurses and midwives generate ideas for research?
- What are some of the challenges that nurses and midwives might face in undertaking research?
- What strategies could be used to promote research in nursing and midwifery practice?

QUESTIONS FOR PERSONAL REFLECTION

- What have you learnt about doing research while working through this chapter?
- Based on your own philosophical beliefs, can you relate more to quantitative or to qualitative approaches?

USEFUL WEB RESOURCES

Australian and New Zealand Clinical Trials Registry <www.anzctr.org.au>

REFERENCES AND FURTHER READING

Alabdulaziz, H., Moss, C. & Copnell, B., 2017, 'Paediatric nurses' perceptions and practices of family-centred care in Saudi hospitals: A mixed methods study', *International Journal of Nursing Studies*, vol. 69, pp. 66–77.

Cresswell, J.W. & Plano-Clark, V.L., 2018, *Designing and Conducting Mixed-Methods Research*, 3rd edn, Thousand Oaks, CA: Sage.

Doyle, L., Brady, A.M. & Byrne, G., 2009, 'An overview of mixed methods research', *Journal of Research in Nursing*, vol. 14, no. 2, pp. 175–185.

Fawcett, B. & Pockett, R., 2015, *Turning Ideas into Research: Theory, design and practice*, London: Sage.

Grant, B. & Giddings, L.S., 2002, 'Making sense of methodologies: A paradigm framework for the novice researcher', *Contemporary Nurse*, vol. 13, no. 1, pp. 10–28.

Miller, W.R., 2010, 'Qualitative research findings as evidence: Utility in nursing practice', *Clinical Nurse Specialist*, vol. 24, no. 4, pp. 191–193, doi: 10.1097/NUR.0b013e3181e36087.

Sharma, T., Bamford, M. & Dodman, D., 2015, 'Person-centred care: An overview of reviews', *Contemporary Nurse*, vol. 51, nos 2–3, pp. 107–120.

Taylor, B. & Francis, K., 2013, *Qualitative Research in the Health Sciences: Methodologies, methods and processes*, Abingdon: Routledge.

Timmins, F., 2015, 'Disseminating nursing research', *Nursing Standard*, vol. 29, no. 48, pp. 34–39.

World Medical Association, 2013, *Declaration of Helsinki: Ethical principles for medical research involving human subjects*, <www.wma.net/policies-post/wma-declaration-of-helsinki-ethical-principles-for-medical-research-involving-human-subjects/>.

CHAPTER 4

Understanding quantitative research approaches

LEARNING OBJECTIVES

After working through this chapter, you should be able to:

- define the term *quantitative research*
- describe benefits of quantitative research for nursing and midwifery practice
- outline the characteristics of experimental and non-experimental research designs
- outline approaches to sampling in quantitative research
- outline the key concepts of descriptive and inferential data analysis
- describe approaches to ensuring validity and reliability in quantitative research.

KEY TERMS AND CONCEPTS

Bias, case-control study, central tendency, cohort study, confidence intervals, confounder, cross-sectional study, data analysis, deductive, descriptive design, descriptive statistics, dispersion, experimental design, hypothesis, inferential statistics, intervention, measurement scales, non-experimental design, normal distribution, probability, quantitative, quasi-experiment, randomised controlled trial, reliability, sampling, skewed distribution, survey, validity, variable

CASE STUDY OVERVIEW

Stephanie and Peter are nurse unit managers in different wards in the hospital mentioned in the previous chapter. As discussed, the hospital has a strong commitment to person-centred care. Stephanie is not sure of the extent to which person-centred care is practised in her ward and thinks it would be a good idea to find out, as a baseline for further action.

Peter, on the other hand, is sure that the nursing care provided in his ward is not as person-centred as it could be; he wants to investigate whether a nurse education program will improve the care. Both these concerns are appropriately addressed using quantitative approaches.

CHAPTER INTRODUCTION

In the previous chapter, we introduced the concept of quantitative research as one of the basic approaches to undertaking research and generating new knowledge, concerned with measuring concepts of interest, testing theories and ultimately predicting outcomes. In this chapter, we will explore this approach in greater detail. We will examine the various ways of undertaking quantitative research—called *designs*—and the kinds of questions they are used to answer. We will also look more closely at how steps in the research process—selecting participants and collecting and analysing data—are undertaken in quantitative approaches.

What is quantitative research?

As we saw in the previous chapter, **quantitative research** is concerned with numbers—measuring, identifying relationships, explaining and ultimately predicting phenomena through the testing of theories. This is known as a **deductive approach**. Quantitative research methods originated in the so-called hard sciences, such as physics and chemistry, and have been adapted for use in researching people. The beliefs and values of those sciences dominate the way we do this sort of research. Quantitative researchers are concerned with 'facts', assuming there is only one reality, or *truth*. In order to discover the *true* answer, all external influences, including the presence of the researcher, must be minimised; thus, the researcher maintains an objective approach. Often, researchers will distance themselves as much as possible from the research process in order to achieve this. The people they research are often called *subjects*, which emphasises this objectivity, although many researchers argue

quantitative research
a research approach, largely deductive, that emphasises objective measurement of information and its numerical analysis

deductive approach
a research approach involving developing and testing a hypothesis

against this terminology. For quite a long time, quantitative research was the only approach accepted in nursing and midwifery (Beyea & Slattery 2013). While this view has changed, the approach is still highly relevant for answering many of the questions of concern to nursing and midwifery practice.

Quantitative designs

The aims of quantitative research can be to describe or explore something of interest, to examine associations between variables or to identify cause-and-effect relationships. In health care, cause-and-effect relationships that we are interested in include causes of disease and the effectiveness of our practices in achieving the aims of the care we provide, which might be prevention or cure of disease, reduction of symptoms, prevention of adverse events, patient satisfaction and so on. A number of research designs have been developed to answer questions relating to these aims. Broadly speaking, these designs can be categorised as either *experimental* or *non-experimental*. Non-experimental designs are often termed *observational* (which should not be confused with observation as a means of collecting data). Experimental designs are specifically focused on identifying cause-and-effect relationships. In this chapter's case study, Peter's question would be ideally answered using an experimental design, as he is interested in whether an education program results in, or causes, an improvement in person-centred care. Non-experimental designs can be used to simply describe phenomena of interest or to examine associations. Stephanie's question is suited to a non-experimental design, as she is interested in describing and measuring the current situation, without manipulating it in any way. Sometimes, cause-and-effect relationships can be inferred from non-experimental research findings, but we must be cautious in making such inferences. A comparison of quantitative research designs is provided in Table 4.1.

Experimental designs

The chief difference between experimental and non-experimental designs is the presence of an **intervention**. Here, intervention has a very precise

TABLE 4.1 Comparison of quantitative designs

Designs	Intervention	Control group	Participant randomisation
Experimental			
RCT	Yes	Yes	Yes
1-group pre-post	Yes	No	N/A
2-group pre-post	Yes	Yes	No
2-group non-parallel	Yes	Yes	No
Non-experimental			
Cohort	No	Yes	No
Case-control	No	Yes	No
Cross-sectional, correlational	No	Occurs by chance, not actively sought	No
Descriptive	No	No	N/A

definition. It is a procedure or practice that is administered or managed by the researchers. The details of the procedure are tightly managed and controlled to ensure that the subjects, or participants, experience it in exactly the same way. For example, researchers might be interested in whether vitamin D supplements can reduce the incidence of osteoporosis. In an experimental study, all participants would receive the same dose of the same preparation of the vitamin, the same number of doses per day, perhaps even taken at the same time of day, for the same duration. Hence, vitamin D supplementation would be the intervention. If the researchers simply studied the general public, who chose for themselves whether or not to take vitamin D, how much to take, when to take it and for how long—in other words, the researchers had no control over its ingestion—then it would not be an intervention, and the researchers would simply be observing the effects (hence, it would be an observational, or non-experimental, study).

intervention
a procedure to which research participants are exposed by the researchers rather than by their own choice; the procedure is managed and controlled by the researchers

Randomised controlled trial or true experiment

The best design for establishing cause-and-effect relationships is the *true experiment*, the classic version of
which is the randomised controlled trial (RCT). You may
remember that in the evidence hierarchy in Chapters 1
and 2 this was ranked highest of the single study designs.
This is because it provides the best assurance that the
outcome of a study (in the above example, incidence
of osteoporosis) is due to the intervention (vitamin D
supplementation) and not to some other influencing
factor, known as a **confounder**. There are several factors
that could influence a person's susceptibility to osteoporosis: age, family history, calcium intake, diet and
amount of exercise, for instance. There are three essential
elements of an RCT:

randomised controlled trial
or **true experiment**
research design that is the most
reliable in establishing cause-and-
effect relationships, requiring the
presence of an intervention, a control
group, and random allocation to the
experimental and the control groups;
also known as RCT

confounder
a factor not related to an intervention
that can influence the outcome being
studied

1 **Intervention** An intervention, as already defined, which is administered to one group of participants (who may be called the *experimental*,
   or *study*, group).
2 **Control group** This is another recruited group, but it does not
   receive the intervention. It should be similar in every other way to the
   experimental group.
3 **Random allocation** The participants are allocated randomly to
   either the experimental or the control group. The aim of this process
   is to achieve even distribution of potential confounders (including
   ones we may not know about) between the two groups.

Importantly, the two groups participate in the study concurrently;
therefore, the design is sometimes referred to as a *two-group parallel RCT*.
The significance of this is that if any changes occur during the study
period, it is highly likely that both groups will be affected in the same
way. Randomisation can be made even more precise by a complex strategy
called *stratified randomisation*, when known confounders are taken into
account. You may come across this term in research reports, but it is not
important to understand it at this stage.

An additional level of rigour in an RCT can be obtained by a process called **blinding**, or **masking**, which means that the group assignment is concealed, for the duration of the study, from the participants, the researchers, anyone who might be making decisions that could affect the outcome, or all of these. In *single blinding*, the participants do not know which group they have been allocated to; this is usually achieved by giving a placebo (such as a sugar pill instead of vitamin D in the above example) to the control group. In *double blinding*, both the participants and the researchers remain unaware of the allocation. This minimises any risk of the researchers treating one group differently, either intentionally or otherwise, to influence the outcome. In clinical research, other people may be able to influence the outcome and should also be unaware of the group allocation. In the above example, for instance, the participants may have nutritionists advising them on their diet; the nutritionists may encourage one group to consume more calcium-containing foods than the other, which could interfere with the results. With some interventions, however, blinding is not possible. In our case study, for instance, Peter wants to test the effectiveness of a nurse education program, and it will be obvious to nurses whether or not they have participated in such a program.

blinding or **masking**
concealment of group allocation from study participants, researchers, others involved in the research, or all three

RCTs do have some disadvantages. They usually require a lot of oversight by the researchers to ensure the procedures are strictly followed, which can be very costly. Other resources can be required too. The researchers need to have sufficient expertise themselves to be able to design and carry out the study, or have expertise available through consultation (for example, statisticians). In some situations, it is not feasible to randomise participants. To return to our case study, if Peter were to conduct an RCT in his ward, he would randomly assign half the participating staff to receive the educational program, while the other half would be randomly assigned not to receive it. However, the two groups would be working side by side; if the members of the control group saw the experimental group practising differently, they might change their behaviour also, in spite of not having received the education. This is known as **contamination** of the two groups.

contamination
a situation where members of a study control group are exposed to the intervention

If the outcome that Peter wants to measure involves the effect on patients, this would be even more problematic, as patients are likely to be cared for by nurses from both groups.

Another form of RCT is the **cluster randomised controlled trial**. This is designed to overcome the problems described in Peter's situation, where it would be very difficult to have the experimental and control groups in the same environment. In this type of study, the unit of randomisation is not the individual participant but a group of participants—in health care, wards or even entire hospitals are often used as groups. In Peter's case, if the hospital where he works is large enough and has several wards similar to his, he could carry out the study by randomising the wards to the experimental and control groups. If the number of available wards is too small, he could recruit similar wards to his from a number of hospitals, again randomly assigning the wards to the two groups. Cluster RCTs are much more difficult to conduct than other studies, usually needing a lot of resources, including financial, and often larger sample sizes than a simple RCT. It is not usually an option for a small research team.

> **cluster randomised controlled trial**
> a randomised controlled trial where the unit of randomisation is not the individual participant but a group of participants

Quasi-experimental designs

If a true experiment is not possible, then a **quasi-experimental design** is the preferred option. This means that either there is no control group or there is a control group but the allocation is not done randomly. These designs are more prone to the effects of confounders and are therefore not considered as rigorous as RCTs.

> **quasi-experimental design**
> an experimental study design where there is no control group, or allocation is not performed randomly

Peter could carry out a quasi-experimental study just with the staff on his ward. He would first measure the level of person-centred care that is currently being delivered. He would then carry out the education program. Following this, he would measure person-centred care again to see if there was a difference from the first measurement. This is sometimes called a **pre-post test**. In this case, there is only one group, so there is no group to compare the results against. Any changes in nurses' practice could

> **pre-post test**
> a study design where measurements are performed before and after an intervention

be due to the education program, but they could also be due to other factors; for example, nurses might have become interested in the topic when the first set of measurements was taken and obtained information themselves on which to base their practice. For this reason, this is considered the weakest of the quasi-experimental designs.

Peter could strengthen the design by including a control group. He could do this by measuring person-centred care on another, similar ward in the hospital where nurses did not participate in the education program. If nurses' practice in this ward did not change, while practice in his own ward, where nurses had participated in the program, did change, Peter could be more confident in attributing the change to the education program and not some confounding factor. However, because the nurses would not have been randomly allocated to either receive the education or not, he could not rule out the possibility that other factors had influenced the outcome. In this situation, the two groups would be studied at the same time, or in parallel, so there would be no confounding effect of different time periods.

Another quasi-experimental design—probably the commonest in clinical research—is known as the *two-group non-randomised non-parallel design*. In it, the outcome of interest is measured in one group, usually patients, exposed to current standard practice; this group functions as the control group. The intervention is then introduced as a change in practice, and the outcome is measured in another group, which is exposed to the new practice. In our case study, Peter could use this design if his outcome related to patients—for instance, patient satisfaction with nursing care. For this, he would measure satisfaction in a group of patients receiving care from nurses who had not been educated in person-centred care. He would then introduce the education program and measure satisfaction in another group of patients, receiving care from nurses who had been educated.

All the designs described in this section are subject to the influence of confounding factors, although the factors themselves vary between designs. Therefore, researchers—and users of research—need to be cautious in attributing any change in the outcome to the effect of the intervention. Hence, quasi-experimental designs are considered weaker than true experiments and are lower in the evidence hierarchy.

Non-experimental designs

Non-experimental designs are characterised by the lack of an intervention. They produce a lower level of evidence than experimental designs. However, sometimes the amount of evidence from non-experimental studies provides a compelling argument for a causative relationship. One example is the link between smoking and lung cancer. The evidence for this link was derived entirely from non-experimental designs, because it is impossible to test using experimental studies as people cannot be forced to smoke. In this case, the evidence was enhanced by laboratory research, which identified the mechanism by which smoking can lead to lung cancer. In the absence of this knowledge, we would still have to say that lung cancer is *associated with*, rather than *caused by*, smoking.

The simplest non-experimental designs are called **descriptive** or *exploratory*. As their names suggest, they are used when researchers simply want to describe and quantify a concept of interest. In our case study, Stephanie would use a descriptive design to measure person-centred care in her ward. She could do this in a number of ways, such as surveying nurses to ask about their practice or observing nurses to see how often they carried out certain practices; we will discuss this in more detail later in the chapter when we consider data collection.

descriptive quantitative design
a non-experimental quantitative study design in which the aim is to describe and quantify a concept of interest; sometimes called an exploratory design

Non-experimental designs can also be used to examine associations between the outcome of interest and other factors; when this is the intent they may be called **correlational designs**. For instance, Stephanie might be interested in whether nurses who have a postgraduate qualification practise person-centred care more than those who do not, or whether there are differences in practice between male and female nurses. She cannot control nurses' gender or their prior education, and therefore she cannot say that any difference she finds is caused by the factor; she can only say there is an association between the factor and the outcome. For this study, Stephanie would collect the data at a specific point in time and once only from each participant, making this a **cross-sectional design**. It is considered the weakest design in terms of establishing associations.

correlational design
a non-experimental study design in which the aim is to investigate associations between the outcome of interest and other factors

cross-sectional design
a non-experimental study design where data are collected at one specific point in time

cohort design
a non-experimental study design
where participants (the cohort) are
studied over a period of time

case-control design
a non-experimental study design
where a group of participants with a
certain condition (cases) is studied
alongside a similar group of people
without the condition (control)

Two non-experimental correlational designs are **cohort** and **case-control designs**. Both are intended to examine associations and are considered more robust than cross-sectional studies, because researchers have more control over the selection of participants and the study conditions. Originally, the designs were developed in epidemiological research, to examine potential risk factors for diseases, and they have been adapted for use in clinical research. To describe these designs, we will return to the example given earlier in this chapter, that of a potential association between vitamin D supplementation and prevention of osteoporosis.

To conduct a cohort study, researchers would recruit a group of people (a cohort is, technically, a naturally occurring group—for example, people born in the same year or living in a certain area) who did not have osteoporosis and had not begun taking dietary supplements. The researchers would follow them over a period of time; they would ask them at regular intervals whether they were taking vitamin D, and they would record who developed osteoporosis. At the end of the study, they would calculate whether there was any difference in the incidence of osteoporosis between those who had taken the supplements and those who had not. A case-control study works in reverse. Researchers would find a group of people who had osteoporosis (cases) and ask them whether they had ever taken vitamin D supplements. They would then find another, similar group of people (controls) who did not have osteoporosis and ask them the same question. Again, they would then calculate whether there was a difference in the incidence of the disease. In both these designs, it would be difficult to attribute any reduction in osteoporosis directly to taking vitamin D—to say that taking vitamin D *caused* the reduction. Taking vitamin D could be part of a general lifestyle (healthy diet, exercise and so on) that would protect against osteoporosis.

Developing a research question

In quantitative approaches, the research question is usually precise and much narrower than in qualitative approaches. In Chapter 3, we looked

ACTIVITY 4.1 Comparing quantitative research designs

1 Search for two research reports on a topic of your choice that have used different quantitative designs.
2 Read the papers carefully.

Questions for consideration

- How is the research question or aim expressed in each report?
- What are the differences between the papers in how they report the methods used?
- Are there any differences in the reporting of the findings?
- Is either of the designs easier to understand as reported in the article? Why?
- What are the implications of each article for your own practice?

at examples of broad questions that related to concerns around person-centred care. These questions would need further refinement for a quantitative study. The wording of the question should be congruent with the study design. For example, if Peter were proposing to undertake an RCT in a medical-surgical ward, his question could be *Do medical-surgical nurses who have undertaken a targeted education program practise person-centred care more frequently than nurses who have not?* If, on the other hand, he were to propose a one-group pre-post study, his question could be *Does the level of person-centred care delivered by medical-surgical nurses increase after undertaking a targeted education program?* As Stephanie is planning a descriptive study, her question could be broader—for example, *How frequently do nurses practise person-centred care in a medical ward?*

An important step in planning a quantitative study is to define the concepts in the research topic and how they will be addressed in the research; this is called *operationalising* the concepts and is usually necessary even with an apparently simple concept. If the concept were hypertension, for instance, we would need to define exactly what level of blood pressure constituted hypertension and which measurement (systolic, diastolic or mean) we were interested in. In our case study, person-centred care is a very broad concept, and both Peter and Stephanie will have to decide how they are going to work with the concept in order to conduct research. They may decide to focus on an actual process of person-centred care, demonstrated through nurses' behaviours. In that case, they will need to work out what behaviours are person centred and what are not, and whether they will focus on all or some of these. They may decide that nurses' attitudes are a good predictor of their practice and focus on measuring those. Alternatively, they may decide to focus on an outcome of person-centred care. This may be a general outcome, such as patient satisfaction with care, or something very specific, such as length of hospital stay, as in the study by Olsson et al. (2016). Thus, the research question could be refined even further once the operationalisation of the concepts had been completed.

As we have seen, the focus in quantitative research is on measuring concepts of interest. Any measured concept or characteristic that can vary in a study is called a **variable**. The actual measurements that can be obtained for a variable are termed its *values*. For example, the variable eye colour can have the values brown, blue, green and grey. The outcome of interest—in this case, person-centred care, however we choose to operationalise it—is called the **dependent variable**. If we are interested in investigating the influence of a specific factor on the outcome, whether or not it is an intervention, it is called the **independent variable**. When the aim of a study is to examine relationships between variables, the research question is usually framed as a **hypothesis**, a statement about the assumed relationship, which the researcher can then test. The scientific method requires that this statement be framed in the negative: this is termed the *null hypothesis*. In Peter's experimental study, the null hypothesis could be *There will be no difference in the practice of person-centred care between nurses who have undertaken an education program and those who have not.* The study should be designed in such a way that the null hypothesis can be disproved (if in fact it is not correct). The *alternative hypothesis* is the opposite of the null hypothesis. The possibilities if the null hypothesis is wrong are twofold:

variable
any measured concept or characteristic that can vary in a study

dependent variable
the outcome of interest in a quantitative study

independent variable
a specific factor that could influence the study outcome

hypothesis
a statement about assumed variable relationships that can be tested

person-centred care could be better if nurses have undertaken an education program, or it could be worse. The most scientific approach is to allow—and therefore test—for either of these possibilities. Therefore, the most appropriate alternative hypothesis would be *There is a difference in the practice of person-centred care by nurses who have and nurses who have not undertaken an education program*. This is called a *non-directional hypothesis*, because it does not privilege one possibility over the other.

The next important step is to determine how the variables of interest will be measured. In quantitative research, we talk of measuring all variables, even non-numeric ones. In a broad sense, how variables are measured depends to a large extent on how we want to analyse the data to answer the research question. In Peter's study, he needs to be able to compare the level of person-centred care delivered by nurses at two points in time. To do this, he must reduce the dependent variable—person-centred care delivered by every nurse in the study—to a single numerical value. Therefore, he needs to find a tool that will enable him to do this. We will look at this further when discussing data collection. His independent variable—the education program—is simply measured as either having or not having been undertaken. The ways in which we can measure variables, whether numerical or not, are called *measurement scales*. These scales are:

- **Categorical or nominal** The values of variables represent a classification or group membership. Examples of variables include gender, hair colour, presence or absence of disease, and participation or non-participation in an education program. There is no logical order to differences between the values.
- **Ordinal** The values are ordered (ranked), but the differences cannot be quantified. Variables may be numerical (such as the order in which people finish a race or the ranking of people taking part in a contest) or non-numerical (such as army ranks).
- **Interval** Differences between values correspond to real, meaningful, consistent differences in the phenomenon being measured. In these variables, there is no *natural zero*; that is, a value of 0 does not represent absence of the entity being measured. Examples include temperature in degrees Celsius and the year of an occurrence: 0 degrees Celsius

does not indicate an absence of temperature, and the year 0 is not the point at which time commenced. What is more, this measurement is not subject to multiplication or division; 200 degrees Celsius is not twice as hot as 100 degrees Celsius, for instance.

- **Ratio** Variables that can be measured on the ratio scale are similar to interval variables in that differences between values are meaningful and consistent, but these variables do have a *natural zero*, indicating absence of the entity (for example, length, duration, weight), and can be multiplied and divided; 10 centimetres is twice as long as 5 centimetres, for instance.

Researchers need to understand these scales, as they largely dictate how data are analysed. The scales are considered as an ascending hierarchy, increasing in complexity from nominal to ratio. The more complex the scale, the more sophisticated the analysis that can be undertaken.

RESEARCH EXAMPLE 4.1 Using a quasi-experimental design with person-centred care as an intervention

Person-centred care is embedded in healthcare philosophy, but what effect does it have on patient outcomes? Olsson et al. (2016) set out to answer this question in patients undergoing hip replacements. Patients were recruited from orthopaedic departments in two hospitals. The first group of patients, recruited between September 2010 and March 2011, received standard care; they formed the control group. Standard care consisted of standardised information, given to them in written and verbal form, about their surgery and what they could expect. The second group of patients, recruited between December 2011 and November 2012, formed the experimental group. The intervention that this group received comprised information tailored to their specific needs, through forming a partnership with a specialist nurse, and participation in formulating a personalised healthcare plan. The researchers found that in the experimental group, vulnerable patients (defined as those with low coping ability, high fear of movement or both) had a shorter length of hospital stay than similar patients in the control group.

L.-E. Olsson, E. Hansson & I. Ekman, 2016, 'Evaluation of person-centred care after hip replacement: A controlled before and after study on the effects of fear of movement and self-efficacy compared to standard care', *BMC Nursing*, vol. 15, no. 53, doi: 10.1186/s12912-016-0173-3.

Questions for consideration
- What features of this study design make it a quasi-experiment rather than a true experiment?
- Why might the researchers have opted to use this design rather than a true experimental design?
- How might the findings be applied to nursing practice?

RESEARCH EXAMPLE 4.2 Using a descriptive quantitative design to study woman-centred midwifery care

Emotionally traumatic birth experiences can have long-lasting effects for women, even leading to post-traumatic stress disorder. Providing woman-centred obstetric and midwifery care can help to identify women at risk of, and may help to prevent, a traumatic birth. Hollander et al. (2017) surveyed 2192 women who had suffered emotional trauma during childbirth, to identify the details of the experience, the women's views on the causes of their trauma, what their caregivers could have done to prevent it and what they themselves would have liked to have done differently. They also administered a number of established questionnaires concerning coping, stress and social support. Women were recruited by invitations placed on a Facebook page set up for the study, Twitter, a study website and other social media. The survey was electronic. The researchers found that women attributed their trauma to multiple causes. The six most commonly cited were loss or lack of control (54.6 per cent), fear for their baby (49.9 per cent), high pain intensity (47.4 per cent), poor communication by caregivers (43.7 per cent), long duration of delivery (37.9 per cent) and lack of practical or emotional support from caregivers (35.6 per cent). Better communication, including listening to the mother, and better support, were identified as the strategies caregivers could have used to prevent the trauma. Poor communication and support were less likely to be cited by mothers who had been cared for by midwives than by those cared for by obstetricians.

M.H. Hollander, E. van Hastenberg, J. van Dillen, M.G. van Pampus, E. de Miranda & C.A.I. Stramrood, 2017, 'Preventing traumatic childbirth experiences: 2192 women's perceptions and views', *Archives of Women's Mental Health*, vol. 20, no. 4, pp. 515–523, doi: 10.1007/s00737-017-0729-6.

Questions for consideration
- What do you consider to be the strengths and weaknesses of this study design?
- What are the implications of the study for midwives?

Sampling and sample size

The aim of sampling in quantitative research is to select participants who will be representative of the population from which they are drawn; that is, the characteristics that are important to the study should be the same in the sample and the population. The likelier this representativeness is, the more confident researchers can be that the results of the research can be applied (generalised) to the population. Sampling methods can be divided into two categories: *probability* and *non-probability* methods. Probability sampling is most likely to achieve a representative sample and is intended to give every member of the population an equal chance of being selected. The strategies are outlined below.

Probability sampling

- **Simple random sampling** In this method, a random-number generator, usually in the form of computer software, is used to select the required number of participants from the population. There is no consideration of any specific characteristics.

- **Stratified random sampling** This method divides the population according to one or more characteristics, and a random sample is drawn from each. It is used to ensure proportional representation of a characteristic; for instance, a population of nurses could be stratified into male and female. As males make up around 10 per cent of the nursing workforce, a similar percentage could be selected to be in the sample.

  probability sampling
  sampling based on random selection

- **Cluster random sampling** Here, the selection is of groups rather than of individuals; for example, a random selection of hospitals could be chosen for people within them to be involved in a study.

- **Systematic sampling** In this method, the participants are chosen not at random but according to a specific schedule; for example, if you were conducting research in women who had recently given birth, you might choose every third mother admitted to a postnatal ward.

Non-probability sampling

- **Convenience sampling** In this method, people are approached because they are readily accessible, and they self-select to take part. People responding to a survey usually constitute a convenience sample. People who feel particularly strongly about a topic or have extreme views may be more likely to take part than other members of the population and so are less likely to be representative.

  non-probability sampling
  sampling that does not involve random selection

- **Quota sampling** The intention in this method is to generate a sample with the same proportion of a characteristic as occurs in the population. Again, people self-select to take part, but they are accepted only until the quota is filled. To use the example of male and female nurses, male nurses who came forward would be accepted until the required number to form 10 per cent of the sample size was reached.

- **Purposive sampling** This method involves hand-picking people with specific characteristics. It is rarely used in quantitative studies.

The number of participants needed for a quantitative study is usually determined before the study commences. In a descriptive study with a convenience sample, the sample size may be simply a pragmatic consideration—the number that can reasonably be expected to take part. The number required to provide reasonable representation of the population can be calculated. In experimental studies, particularly RCTs, the sample size must be sufficient to enable detection of a true difference between the groups and is always calculated beforehand. This notion is rather complex but relates to the statistical concept of probability—that is, if we find there is a difference in the outcome between the experimental and control groups, we have to determine whether this occurred by chance or because of a real effect of the intervention. In analysing the data (which we will look at in more detail presently), we calculate, using a statistical test, the probability, or likelihood, of the difference occurring by chance. If the sample size is too small, the test result will suggest the finding occurred by chance. The likelihood that the test will correctly indicate a real effect of the intervention is called the **power** of the study.

power
the likelihood of a test correctly indicating a real effect of an intervention due to sufficient sample size

Collecting data

Any of the sources of data described in the previous chapter can be used in quantitative studies. However, the format in which data are collected is very specific. As discussed above, data must be collected so that all variables can be measured in an appropriate way to answer the research question. For example, Stephanie could choose to collect data for her descriptive study by observing nurses in her ward. She would need to decide what specific behaviours by nurses constituted person-centred care or non-person-centred care and then record instances of these behaviours when they were observed. The nurses' activities could thus be quantified.

A specific type of data collection used in quantitative research is the survey, or questionnaire. In quantitative research, surveys usually consist mainly of closed-ended questions; that is, a finite list of answers is provided from which the participants must choose. One particular style of question that is often used in surveys is the **Likert scale** question. A Likert scale is a rating scale on which participants respond to a series of statements. Responses often range from 'Strongly disagree' to 'Strongly agree', or similar terms

Likert scale
a rating scale that allows participants to indicate their level of agreement with presented statements

relevant to the question. Surveys can consist of related but independent questions designed to explore a particular situation. The questions in the survey by Hollander et al. (2017) relating to women's experiences of birth trauma fall into this category. Surveys can also consist of questions that, when taken together, measure a specific entity, such as person-centred care, patient satisfaction or interprofessional collaboration. Developing a survey tool is a complex process with several issues to consider (Blair et al. 2014). It is preferable to see if there is an existing tool suitable for the purpose of a planned survey. This not only saves time and effort; it enables results from studies using the same tool to be compared or data to be combined to enhance knowledge on the topic.

ACTIVITY 4.2 Designing a quantitative study

1 Using the concept of person-centred care, imagine you are planning a quantitative study with the focus on how nursing students understand the concept.
2 Choose one quantitative research design that you could use for the study.
3 Write a short, clear research question that could be answered using your chosen design.

Questions for consideration
- Where would you find the right participants?
- What sampling process would be appropriate for your study?
- How would you go about recruiting participants?
- What data would you need to collect to answer your question?
- How would you collect the data?

Analysing data

Analysis of quantitative data is almost always undertaken using computer software. Some analysis can be performed using a simple spreadsheet program, such as Microsoft Excel, while more complex operations require a dedicated statistical package. There are many of these on the market;

one of the most commonly used, and supported by many institutions, is IBM SPSS. There are two levels of quantitative **data analysis**, known as descriptive and inferential. *Descriptive statistics* are used, as the name suggests, to describe data by summarising them. In a purely descriptive study, this would be the only level of analysis performed. In other studies, it would be the first level of analysis. *Inferential statistics* are used to examine associations between variables and to draw inferences between the sample (in whom the measurements have been taken) and the wider population.

data analysis
the process of analysing collected data to draw conclusions

normal distribution
symmetrical distribution of data with the majority of data points clustered around the centre; when represented graphically it forms a bell-shaped curve

An important concept in data analysis is the **normal distribution**, in which data values, when presented graphically, form a symmetrical bell-shaped curve, with the majority clustered around the centre and the rest tapering out towards both ends (see Figure 4.1). Many large datasets will form this distribution. An asymmetrical distribution, with a longer tail at one end than at the

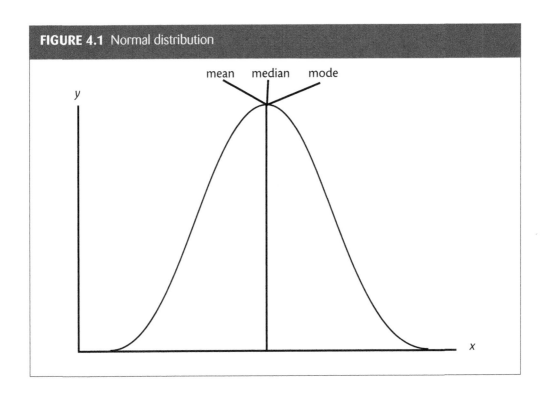

FIGURE 4.1 Normal distribution

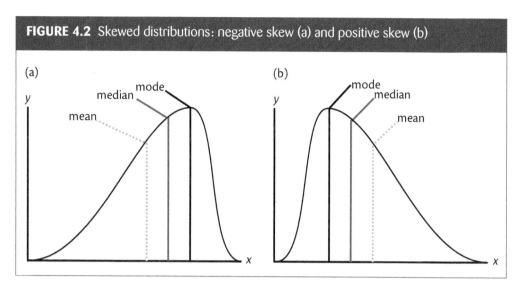

FIGURE 4.2 Skewed distributions: negative skew (a) and positive skew (b)

other, is called a **skewed distribution** (see Figure 4.2). In a positively skewed distribution, the longer tail is to the right, while a negatively skewed distribution has a longer tail to the left. It is important to know whether data are normally distributed or skewed, as different analytic techniques are required for each.

Descriptive statistics

There are two types of measurements that are used to summarise data; they are referred to as **central tendency** and **dispersion**. Central tendency is the tendency of data to cluster around a point towards the middle of the range; this is illustrated in the bell shape of the normal distribution. Central tendency can be measured in the following ways:

skewed distribution
asymmetrical data distribution; when represented graphically the curve has a longer tail at one end than the other

descriptive statistics
measures used to summarise raw data

central tendency
a measure, generally towards the middle of a dataset, around which data points are clustered; potential measures are mean, median and mode

dispersion
a measure of the degree of variability in a dataset; potential measures are variance, standard deviation, range, interquartile range and frequency

- **Mean** The average of a set of numbers, obtained by summing all the values and dividing by the number of values in the dataset.
- **Median** The middle value when the values in a dataset are placed in numerical order; if there is an even number of values, the median is calculated by taking the average of the two middle numbers.
- **Mode** The most frequently occurring value in a dataset.

In a normal distribution, the mean, median and mode are all the same (see Figure 4.1). In a skewed distribution, the mean is pulled away from the median in the direction of the tail (see Figure 4.2) and is therefore less representative of the dataset.

Measures of dispersion tell us about the amount of variation in the data. The measures that can be used are:

- **Frequency** The count of the occurrences of values in a dataset expressed as a number, a percentage or a proportion.
- **Range** The difference between the highest and lowest values in a dataset.
- **Variance** In simple terms, the average of the differences between each individual value and the mean. To make the mathematical calculation possible, each of the values must be squared. This measure is rarely used in practice.
- **Standard deviation** The square root of the variance, in essence correcting for the squaring of values that occurred in calculating the variance. It is nearly always used in preference to the variance.
- **Percentile** The value at or below which lies a certain percentage of values in a distribution. For example, 10 per cent of the distribution will lie below the 10th percentile. (Percentiles are used in clinical practice when tracking growth measures; infants' weight and head circumference and children's height, weight and body mass index are all tracked using percentile charts.) The 25th, 50th and 75th percentiles divide the distribution into quarters and are therefore called the 1st, 2nd and 3rd quartiles (and, of course, the 50th percentile, or 2nd quartile, is also the median, as described above).
- **Interquartile range** The difference between the 1st and 3rd quartiles; also known as IQR.

The measures of central tendency and dispersion are not interchangeable and should be used for specific scales of measurement; these are summarised in Table 4.2. Knowing how the measures are derived can be helpful in understanding their use, but it is no longer necessary to know how to calculate them: any computer program capable of data analysis

TABLE 4.2 Descriptive statistics and when to use them		
Measurement scale	**Central tendency**	**Dispersion**
Nominal (categorical)	Mode	Frequency
Ordinal		
Non-numerical variable	Mode	Frequency
Numerical variable	Median	Range, interquartile range
Interval, ratio		
Normal distribution	Mean	Variance, standard deviation
Skewed distribution	Median	Range, interquartile range

will do this for you. It is more important to be able to interpret them, particularly measures of dispersion. The higher the dispersion, the more variability there is in the data, and hence the less the measure of central tendency represents the sample.

Inferential statistics

Inferential analysis examines associations between variables and provides information on whether results obtained from a study sample can be generalised to the population. The assumption underpinning this is that results may not be replicated exactly if the study were to be undertaken in another sample or if the findings were to be implemented into practice; that is, some variation would be expected. Data can be analysed using a wide variety of statistical tests using statistical software. Which test is used depends on a number of things, including what the researcher wants to know and what scale of measurement applies to the variables. Some of the simpler and more common tests, and the circumstances in which they are used, are listed in Research tip 4.1. It is important that researchers understand what the various tests do and when they are used; the

inferential statistics
tests carried out on data to determine whether the results can be generalised from the sample to the population

ACTIVITY 4.3 Descriptive statistics and measurement scales

The table contains details of final marks and grades obtained by a class of 30 students.

Student code	Status	Gender	Mark	Grade
1	International	M	90	HD
2	Domestic	M	67	C
3	International	F	55	P
4	Domestic	F	55	P
5	International	M	75	D
6	Domestic	F	88	HD
7	International	F	65	C
8	International	F	49	F
9	International	M	57	P
10	International	M	76	D
11	International	F	61	C
12	Domestic	M	82	HD
13	Domestic	F	75	D
14	Domestic	M	71	D
15	Domestic	F	65	C
16	Domestic	F	85	HD
17	Domestic	M	56	P
18	Domestic	M	40	F
19	Domestic	M	67	C
20	Domestic	F	54	P
21	International	F	36	F
22	International	M	65	C
23	International	M	87	HD
24	Domestic	F	52	P
25	Domestic	M	68	C
26	Domestic	F	53	P
27	Domestic	M	77	D
28	International	F	65	C
29	Domestic	M	42	F
30	International	F	72	D

Note: HD high distinction, D distinction, C credit, P pass, F fail

---

Questions for consideration

- What is the appropriate measurement scale for each of the variables: status, gender, mark and grade?
- Calculate the mean, median and mode of the marks.
- From your answers to the above, do you infer that the distribution of marks is normal or skewed? Give reasons for your answer.

---

software cannot make this decision itself. There are two ways of assessing the statistical significance of associations between variables: through **probability** and **confidence intervals**. In older research reports, you are likely to see only probability mentioned, while in some recent reports, you may only see confidence intervals. However, both are often reported.

Probability is the likelihood of a result occurring by chance. It is represented by p or sometimes P, and it is

probability
the likelihood of a result occurring by chance

confidence intervals
parameters between which the true difference between measurements, or effect of an intervention, would lie if it were measured in the whole population

---

RESEARCH TIP 4.1 Common statistical tests and their purposes

Chi square	Compares two categorical variables, each of which has two or more values
T-test	Compares a continuous (ratio or interval) variable between two groups
Analysis of variance	Compares a continuous (ratio or interval) variable between three or more groups; also known as ANOVA
Correlation	Compares two continuous variables when both are measured, not manipulated
Regression	Examines the effect of manipulating one continuous variable (the independent variable) on a continuous outcome variable (the dependent variable)

expressed as a proportion of 1. Its potential range is from an infinitely small number to 1; that is, it can never be 0. To put it another way, we can never be absolutely certain that any finding is not due to chance alone rather than to a real effect of the independent variable. The smaller the number, however, the less likely it is that the finding is due to chance rather than to a real effect. Researchers choose in advance what limit they are prepared to place on this uncertainty; this is termed *statistical significance*, the upper limit of p at which they are prepared to claim their findings are due to a real difference in their data. By convention, the value of $p = 0.05$ is usually chosen; this means there is a 5 in 100, or 5 per cent, likelihood of the results occurring by chance.

As an example, consider Peter's research in our case study. Let us suppose that when he measures nurses' person-centred care before the education program, he finds that the mean score across his sample is 50 per cent; that is, they are practising person-centred care 50 per cent of the time on average. The measure following the program is 65 per cent— an increase of 15 per cent. The statistical test results in a p-value of 0.03. This means there is a 3 per cent probability of the result occurring by chance, which is a small value and below the conventional level of significance. Thus, Peter can reasonably attribute the change in nurses' scores to his education program and not to some random occurrence. On the other hand, if he obtained a p-value of 0.4, this would indicate a 40 per cent probability that the result occurred by chance, and he could not assume that the difference was due to his program.

Confidence intervals provide a more precise way of judging whether findings can be generalised to a population. They indicate what the likely result would be in the population as a whole, or, to put it another way, they give an estimate of the true effect of the independent variable. Any confidence interval can be calculated, but it is conventional to use 95 per cent; that is, we can be 95 per cent confident that the true result lies between the calculated parameters. The wider the confidence interval, the more uncertainty there is in the truth of the findings.

Let us return to the example above, in which Peter finds a 15 per cent increase in person-centred care after his education program. Suppose he calculates the 95 per cent confidence intervals to be 10 and 20: that would mean he can be 95 per cent certain that the true effect of the program was to increase person-centred care somewhere between 10 per cent and 20 per cent. A reader could then judge whether it would be worth implementing the program or not.

Research rigour

In quantitative research, the main evaluation of research rigour is the extent to which it is free from **bias**. Bias has a very specific meaning in quantitative research: it is a systematic error in the way participants are selected, outcomes are measured or data are analysed that leads to results being inaccurate. All research designs are subject to bias to some degree, from various sources, but some are more susceptible than others.

bias
a systematic error in the way participants are selected, outcomes are measured or data are analysed that leads to results being inaccurate

Validity

The validity of research findings is their accuracy. In research designs that examine associations between variables, we distinguish between internal and external validity. **Internal validity** means that the outcome (dependent variable) is associated with or caused by the explanatory or independent variable rather than a confounding factor. **External validity** refers to the extent to which findings can be generalised.

One aspect of research rigour is the accuracy with which variables are measured. When using any type of instrument to take measurements, we need to be certain that it has both validity and reliability. The **validity of an instrument** refers to whether it accurately measures what it is supposed to measure. For instance, a thermometer is a valid instrument of temperature measurement, but if we tried to use it to measure blood pressure, it would be invalid. Survey instruments—questionnaires—work in the same way. If we wanted to use a survey tool to measure an aspect of person-centred care, for example, we would need to make sure it was actually measuring that and not another concept.

internal validity
the ability to attribute the outcome of a research study to the effect of the independent variable and not some other factor

external validity
the ability to generalise the results of a study beyond the study sample

validity of an instrument
the accuracy with which a research instrument or tool measures what it is supposed to measure

Reliability

Reliability is the consistency with which an instrument measures the construct. The same result should be obtained if the measurements are taken repeatedly, so that changes in the measurement represent a real change in what is being measured. To return to the example of the thermometer, we would expect that if we used it to take someone's temperature several times in a short period we would obtain the same result. We expect survey instruments to perform in a similar way. Research reports that have used a survey tool should report on both the validity and the reliability of the tool and how these were established.

reliability
the consistency with which a research instrument measures the construct

---

RESEARCH EXAMPLE 4.3 Tools to measure person-centred care

When conducting a survey using an established tool, it is important to ensure that the tool is fit for the purpose for which it will be used—that it has validity (measures what we want it to measure) and reliability (measures the same concept consistently). A number of tools have been developed to measure person-centred care in a range of environments. Edvardsson and Innes (2010) reviewed the tools that were available to measure the person centredness of care for older people and people with dementia. They identified twelve such tools, most of which had not been used in research since their initial development. They concluded that tool selection was largely dependent on the research question.

D. Edvardsson & A. Innes, 2010, 'Measuring person-centered care: A critical comparative review of published tools', *The Gerontologist*, vol. 50, no. 6, pp. 834–836.

Questions for consideration

- How can articles such as this assist researchers?
- What are the implications of this study for nursing and midwifery practice?

ACTIVITY 4.4 Analysing a quantitative research paper

1 Locate a quantitative research paper on a topic of interest to you.
2 Carefully review the paper, examining the description of the data analysis in the methods section and the reported results.

Questions for consideration
- How were the data analysed?
- Are statistical methods clearly explained and tests named?
- Are p-values or confidence intervals, or both, reported?
- Are the results clear?
- What have the authors reported about validity and/or reliability?
- Have they identified potential sources of bias?
- Do the methods appear sufficiently rigorous to you?
- What do you consider to be the strengths and weaknesses of the report?

Reporting findings

Reports of quantitative research share a very similar structure, whatever research design was used:

- **Background or introduction** This sets out what is already known about the topic and explains why the current research was undertaken.
- **Aim** This is usually phrased as a statement of purpose but may be phrased as a question; either way the intent of the research should be clear. A hypothesis should be included for experimental studies.
- **Methods** This section is particularly important, as this is what is mainly used to judge the rigour of the study. Moreover, the methods should be described in sufficient detail that another researcher could replicate the study. The section should include descriptions of the setting, the sample (including sample size and how it was determined), how participants were recruited, all study procedures, what data were collected and how, and how data were analysed.

- **Results** The findings are presented in this section, often in the form of tables or figures. There should be enough descriptive statistics for readers to judge the similarity between the study participants and the people to whom they would apply the findings. Results of statistical tests should be presented in a standard format without interpretation.

- **Discussion** This section interprets the findings and places them in context, discusses the implications of the results and identifies limitations of the study.

Reporting standards have been developed for a range of research designs (see Research tip 4.2 for examples), and it is expected that all publications will follow them. This enables readers to judge whether the research has been undertaken rigorously and the degree of potential bias. The standards can be accessed through the EQUATOR (Enhancing the Quality and Transparency of Health Research) Network, at <www.equator-network.org>.

RESEARCH TIP 4.2 Reporting standards relevant to quantitative designs

CHEERS	Economic evaluations
CONSORT	RCTs
SQUIRE	Quality improvement studies
STARD	Diagnostic and prognostic studies
STROBE	Observational studies

CHAPTER SUMMARY

Quantitative research is commonly used in nursing and midwifery research. It enables concepts to be quantified, either for purely descriptive purposes or to compare across different situations. It enables exploration of relationships between concepts (variables) and is particularly important in determining the effectiveness of practices and therapeutic interventions. In this chapter, we have explored some of the quantitative designs that can be used to address specific questions and the steps involved in undertaking quantitative research. Data collection for quantitative studies can be carried out in many ways, but the data must be quantifiable for analysis. Data analysis can be descriptive or inferential. The validity of study findings—that is, the degree to which they are free from bias—is an important concept in quantitative research.

CHAPTER REVIEW QUESTIONS

- What is meant by *quantitative research*?
- What are some of the common quantitative designs used in nursing and midwifery research? How do they differ?
- What types of data do quantitative researchers collect?
- What are the main processes for quantitative data analysis?
- How are validity and reliability achieved in quantitative research?

QUESTIONS FOR DISCUSSION

- What are some possible applications for quantitative research in nursing and midwifery practice?
- How can nurses and midwives contribute to quantitative research knowledge and use?
- What are some of the challenges that might be faced in undertaking quantitative research?
- What strategies could be used to promote quantitative research in nursing and midwifery practice?

QUESTIONS FOR PERSONAL REFLECTION

- How could quantitative research be employed to improve nursing or midwifery care?
- What have you learnt about quantitative research while working through this chapter?

USEFUL WEB RESOURCES

Enhancing the Quality and Transparency of Health Research Network <www.equator-network.org>

REFERENCES AND FURTHER READING

Beyea, S.C. & Slattery, M.J., 2013, 'Historical perspectives on evidence-based nursing', *Nursing Science Quarterly*, vol. 26, no. 2, pp. 152–155.

Blair, J., Czaja, R.F. & Blair, E.A., 2014, *Designing Surveys: A guide to decisions and procedures*, 3rd edn, Thousand Oaks, CA: Sage.

Edvardsson, D. & Innes, A., 2010, 'Measuring person-centered care: A critical comparative review of published tools', *The Gerontologist*, vol. 50, no. 6, pp. 834–836.

Field, A., 2013, *Discovering Statistics Using IBM SPSS Statistics*, 4th edn, London: Sage.

Hayat, M.J., 2013, 'Understanding sample size determination in nursing research', *Western Journal of Nursing Research*, vol. 35, no. 7, pp. 943–956.

Hoare, Z. & Hoe, J., 2013, 'Understanding quantitative research', part 2, *Nursing Standard*, vol. 27, no. 18, pp. 48–55.

Hoe, J. & Hoare, Z., 2012, 'Understanding quantitative research', part 1, *Nursing Standard*, vol. 27, nos 15–17, pp. 52–57.

Hollander, M.H., van Hastenberg, E., van Dillen, J., van Pampus, M.G., de Miranda, E. & Stramrood, C.A.I., 2017, 'Preventing traumatic childbirth experiences: 2192 women's perceptions and views', *Archives of Women's Mental Health*, vol. 20, no. 4, pp. 515–523, doi: 10.1007/s00737-017-0729-6.

Olsson, L.-E., Hansson, E. & Ekman, I., 2016, 'Evaluation of person-centred care after hip replacement: A controlled before and after study on the effects of fear of movement and self-efficacy compared to standard care', *BMC Nursing*, vol. 15, no. 53, doi: 10.1186/s12912-016-0173-3.

Pallant, J., 2016, *SPSS Survival Manual: A step by step guide to data analysis using IBM SPSS*, 6th edn, Sydney: Allen & Unwin.

CHAPTER 5

Understanding qualitative research approaches

LEARNING OBJECTIVES

After working through this chapter, you should be able to:

- define the term *qualitative research*
- describe benefits of qualitative research for nursing or midwifery practice
- outline basic approaches to and differences between common qualitative research methodologies
- outline the two main ways by which qualitative data analysis is performed
- discuss strategies for ensuring quality and rigour in qualitative research.

KEY TERMS AND CONCEPTS

Action research, audit trail, case study, confirmability, content analysis, credibility, data saturation, descriptive, discourse analysis, ethnography, fittingness, grounded theory, immersion, inductive, interpretive, methodology, paradigm, participatory research, phenomenology, qualitative, realities, thematic analysis, transferability, triangulation

CASE STUDY OVERVIEW

Jill is the unit manager for a busy medical-surgical unit. The ward has a strong philosophy around delivering person-centred care. However, lately, Jill has observed that nurses in the ward appear to be providing care that is not necessarily person-centred, and she is wondering whether this is related to their understanding of the philosophy and what it means. She wants to understand how the nurses perceive their implementation of person-centred care into their everyday work and whether there are other factors impacting on their abilities to deliver person-centred care. She decides that this kind of study requires a qualitative approach.

CHAPTER INTRODUCTION

In the previous chapter, we explored quantitative methods for generating new knowledge and understandings. With quantitative approaches, the emphasis is on use of measurements and numbers. However, there are other types of data that are equally important for informing practice—that is, qualitative types. Qualitative research entails seeking understandings of human experiences and situations, primarily through using words and text. This chapter focuses on qualitative research and how it applies to nursing and midwifery. One of the challenges in qualitative research is that there are many approaches and positions taken by researchers. While the chapter does not seek to offer insights into all of these, it aims to present an overview of the nature of qualitative research generally, with exploration of a few of the most commonly used approaches.

What is qualitative research?

Qualitative research is popular in nursing and midwifery as it involves close interaction with the people being studied, reflecting the levels of communication and personal interaction involved in professional nursing and midwifery work. It seeks to understand varied human realities and contexts. Qualitative research allows for rich understandings and can lead to development of theories that explain certain situations. Hence, it is well suited to nursing and midwifery practice, as they are both very interactive professions. It can also be useful when little is known about a particular topic and the researcher seeks to understand it better. Sometimes, qualitative research is used in mixed methods research to gain an understanding of a topic for which a quantitative survey can be subsequently developed. Alternatively, qualitative research may be used after a quantitative study to more fully understand the nature of a topic that cannot be explored in depth in a survey.

qualitative research
a research approach, primarily inductive, that seeks to make meaning of human experience

Differences between qualitative and quantitative research

As described in the previous chapter, quantitative research involves measuring and analysing relationships between variables—for example, through frequencies and other statistical analyses. Largely, quantitative research answers What? and How much? questions. On the other hand, qualitative research seeks understandings of processes and situations. It looks at how processes work and how individuals experience them.

The language of qualitative research is different from that of quantitative research and at times can seem overwhelming for a new reader. First, the person is seen as central to the whole process of qualitative research. Therefore, while people may be referred to as a group of *subjects* in quantitative research, in qualitative studies people who participate are known as *participants*. Second, there are multiple viewpoints, or **paradigms**, from which qualitative research is approached. **Interpretive research** attempts to interpret the experiences of people, while **participatory research** aims to work with participants to make change—participation is active—therefore, the relationship between the researcher and participants can differ.

paradigm
a particular viewpoint of the world

interpretive research
qualitative research that seeks to make meaning of a phenomenon

participatory research
qualitative research that actively involves participants in making change

While quantitative research believes there is one answer, or truth, qualitative research reflects the individual nature of human existence and explores social constructions. It believes that there are many ways to view the world and that each person's own truth is relevant and legitimate. Hence, qualitative research assumes multiple ways of seeing something. Consider, for example, patients' experiences of being in hospital: no two patients have completely the same experience, but each experience is real and relevant to the individual patient.

Given the different natures of qualitative research approaches, the data used are also different. Quantitative research is dependent on numbers and mathematical calculations. On the other hand, qualitative research collects mainly words or text. However, it may also draw on other types of data such as pictures and photographs.

Common qualitative approaches

There are many ways to go about qualitative research. The approach chosen is dependent on the research aim and question to be answered and upon the philosophical perspectives of the researcher. Our goal here is not to conduct an exhaustive discussion of each type but to have you appreciate that there are different approaches to conducting qualitative research. This will assist you as you read qualitative studies and try to make sense of them. There are many more qualitative approaches in nursing and midwifery than are covered in this chapter, but commonly used approaches include those discussed below.

Phenomenology

In phenomenology, the research is focused on understanding the meanings in the lived experiences of people in certain situations, or phenomena.

phenomenology
a qualitative research methodology
that examines human lived experience

This draws in the similarities and differences in people's experiences across similar situations. The researcher may *bracket*, or put aside, their own preconceived ideas on a situation. A range of specific approaches has evolved as phenomenology itself has evolved. In this chapter's case study, Jill may choose to use phenomenology to explore the experiences of staff in delivering patient-centred care. Even though she thinks she might know what the issues impacting on this are, she needs to put her own ideas aside and focus on those of her participants. Jill should not let her own preconceived ideas influence the analysis and interpretations of her findings.

Qualitative descriptive research

Sometimes, a researcher may choose to perform qualitative research without a strong philosophical underpinning so will carry out a descrip-

qualitative descriptive research
a qualitative research approach
that seeks to describe a particular
phenomenon

tive qualitative study. This is similar to phenomenology in the way that the researcher seeks to provide a rich description of the topic or issue under study, but the researcher is less concerned with their own role or bias in the study or in the underlying philosophical position. However, the researcher still needs to collect sufficient data to be able to draw sound conclusions. In our case study, if Jill were to employ a descriptive qualitative research approach to understanding the factors impacting on patient-centred care, she might choose to interview a number of staff members and analyse the interviews without a particularly focused approach.

Grounded theory

This approach explores social processes and how they work, by examining interactions between people (Hall et al. 2013). This allows a theory or model to be constructed that shows how processes operate and that is generated from, and grounded in, the data collected. Within grounded theory, there is a range of specific approaches that have evolved as grounded theory itself has evolved. In our case study, if Jill were to take a grounded theory approach, it would look different to that of other qualitative approaches.

grounded theory
a research methodology that examines social processes in order to develop theory

RESEARCH TIP 5.1 Common qualitative approaches used in nursing and midwifery

Action research	Works with individuals or groups to make, implement and evaluate changes (see Chapter 8)
Case study	Examines the complexities of unique stories to explore a particular phenomenon
Discourse analysis	Examines social and political factors that shape the development of certain practices or circumstances
Ethnography	Examines cultural patterns existing in a particular group
Ethnomethodology	Examines the ways in which people feel, understand and explain their world
Grounded theory	Examines social processes and how they work in certain situations
Historical research	Examines the historical development of a particular concept or situation
Narrative research	Explores the experiences of people through the stories they tell
Phenomenology	Examines the lived experiences of individuals in certain situations

Jill would be focusing more on *how* staff actually went about providing patient-centred care in the ward, rather than just describing what happens or their personal experiences.

ACTIVITY 5.1 Exploring a qualitative research approach

1 Choose one qualitative research approach and do some reading about its origins and evolution.
2 Search for one or two research studies that have used that methodology.
3 Summarise the key aspects of the methodology.

Questions for consideration

• How have the researchers in your chosen studies used the methodology?
• Can you think of a study where you could use that particular methodology?

Steps in undertaking a qualitative research study

Qualitative research studies follow similar steps to quantitative studies— that is, identifying a problem or issue, conducting an initial literature review, developing a research question, identifying the population under study, considering the ethical aspects in conducting the study, collecting data, analysing data and then reporting the findings. However, there are some differences in how the research question is framed, the actual ethical considerations and how the data are collected, analysed and reported. (Ethical considerations are covered in more detail in Chapter 7.)

Developing a qualitative research question

Unlike quantitative research, which seeks to quantify or connect cause and effect, qualitative research seeks to understand a particular topic or issue in more depth. Developing a qualitative research question requires great consideration to ensure that it will actually answer the identified problem or issue. A sound research question is clear, specific and able to be researched. Unlike quantitative research questions, qualitative research questions are open ended in nature. The aim is to not limit what might be found and to yield large amounts of textual or observational data. Closed-ended questions do not facilitate the acquisition of such data.

In our case study, Jill wants to understand what staff understand by the concept of person-centred care and what impacts on their ability to deliver such care. Appropriately descriptive qualitative questions might include the following:

- What are nurses' understandings of person-centred care?
- What factors impact on nurses' abilities to deliver person-centred care, and in what ways?
- How do nurses perceive their delivery of person-centred care in the ward?

If Jill wants to use a particular qualitative approach, she may use slightly more refined questions:

- For a phenomenological study, she might ask: *What are the nurses' lived experiences of delivering person-centred care in the ward?*
- If it was a grounded theory study, she might ask: *How do nurses deliver person-centred care in the ward?*
- If she chose a **discourse analysis**, the question might be: *What shapes the way in which nurses deliver patient-centred care in the ward?*

discourse analysis
a research approach that examines social and political factors that shape the development of certain practices or circumstances

---

ACTIVITY 5.2 Exploring person-centred care qualitatively

Imagine you want to explore nursing students' experiences of delivering person-centred care in their clinical placements. Write a short, clear research question that could be asked for each of the following research approaches:
- descriptive qualitative
- phenomenology
- grounded theory.

It is important for the question to align with the type of qualitative approach used. The goal is to keep the question broad, in order to access the types of data required. Activity 5.2 provides an opportunity to develop research questions aligned to a specific approach.

Collecting qualitative data

There are many approaches to collecting qualitative data, including interviews, observations of people in their natural environments, written text sources such as newspapers, documents and records, photographs and other pictures, and social media posts. For example, a phenomenological researcher wanting to understand the patient experience of living with chronic back pain might choose to do one-on-one interviews with patients to record their individual experiences. The grounded theory researcher might choose to explore the processes by which the person copes with their chronic pain, and then develop a model by which patients live with such conditions, so might use a combination of interviews and observations of people in their homes. Common data collection methods in qualitative research include the following:

- **Interviews** Most often, interviews are performed one to one, that is, between the researcher and the person being researched. The researcher may use very structured or semi-structured interview questions, depending on the underlying research approach being taken. Interviews are usually audio-recorded, transcribed verbatim (word for word) and then analysed.
- **Focus groups** These are a type of interview conducted with a group of people at the same time. They give participants the opportunity to explore collective experiences through sharing and building on ideas. Focus groups normally contain from two to ten participants. Like individual interviews, they are usually audio-recorded and transcribed later for analysis. However, there may also be an observer in the room taking field notes—for example, about the interaction of participants.

- **Participant observation** This involves observing participants in the research setting; the researcher usually takes field notes recording their observations for later analysis.
- **Photovoice** This is a newer, but increasingly popular, qualitative research approach, particularly in participatory research, such as action research. It employs the use of photographs to present viewpoints from participants' unique worlds.
- **Surveys** Qualitative survey responses commonly seek open-ended responses rather than closed-ended responses that can be analysed using statistics.

RESEARCH TIP 5.2 Potential data sources for qualitative research

Audio	Interviews, focus groups, podcasts
Electronic	Internet, social media posts
Visual	Pictures, video footage, photographs, observation
Written	Newspapers, magazines, reports, documents, diaries, letters

---

In our case study, it is evident that Jill has a number of options for collecting the data needed to answer her research question. She could do individual interviews, run focus groups with staff, observe staff in their practice or ask them to document their ideas about patient-centred care delivery. Therefore, Jill will need to be clear about her research approach and how best to answer her research question. What would you suggest?

ACTIVITY 5.3 Planning qualitative research

Choose one of the research questions you designed in Activity 5.2.

Questions for consideration
- How might you source the data needed to answer the question?
- Who might your participants be?
- What might be the best method or methods to access the data?

Sourcing research participants and collecting data

Unlike quantitative research, qualitative studies use small samples. Participants for these studies are usually chosen through convenience, or **purposive sampling**. The qualitative researcher does not seek to generalise their findings to other populations, and they look for people who can provide the specific information that will help them answer their research question and understand the phenomenon they are studying.

In seeking out suitable participants, qualitative researchers often use an approach known as **snowball sampling**. This involves using recommendations for suitable participants from people already participating in the research: the sampling rolls on like a snowball.

Theoretical sampling is a technique used in grounded theory approaches. The process of sampling continues until the theory being generated is completed. It is used 'to determine where, when and how to collect further data that will inform the developing theory' (Mills et al. 2014, p. 113).

Qualitative research does not have tight sample-size boundaries such as those associated with quantitative methods. At the point of **data saturation**—when the researcher is not obtaining any new data or new insights into the phenomenon being studied—they need to make the decision to stop collecting data. This is a

purposive sampling
a sampling approach involving purposefully selecting research participants

snowball sampling
a sampling method where current participants in a study recommend future potential participants

theoretical sampling
a sampling technique used in grounded theory, involving sampling until the generated theory is complete

data saturation
the point in qualitative data collection where no new data are being obtained

---

ACTIVITY 5.4 Collecting qualitative data

Choose one of the research questions you designed in Activity 5.2.

Questions for consideration
- Where would you find the right participants to provide data for the research?
- What sampling processes would you employ?
- Where would be the best place to collect the data?
- When would you stop the data collection process?

particularly important concept, as failure to achieve data saturation may negatively impact on the overall conclusions drawn from the study and its potential validity (Fusch & Ness 2015).

Returning to our chapter case study, let's consider how Jill decides to proceed with her qualitative research. Following a great deal of consideration, Jill decides to undertake a descriptive qualitative study to really understand the staff perceptions and understandings of person-centred care. Her research aim is to examine their understandings of person-centred care. In line with that, she develops her research question: *What are nurses' understandings of person-centred care?* Jill then decides that the most appropriate data collection method is semi-structured interview. Her **interview schedule** contains two key guiding questions but allows sufficient space for discussion to proceed in other directions. The key questions are:

interview schedule
key questions used for guiding a research interview

- What do you understand by the term *person-centred care*?
- How do you perceive that person-centred care is provided in your clinical setting?

Jill opts to employ purposive sampling, as she plans to target a specific group of participants—that is, the staff working on the ward. She realises that there may not be enough participants on her ward to enable her to achieve data saturation so considers employing snowball sampling, with her initial participants recommending other potential participants.

Managing and analysing qualitative data

When and how the process of data analysis begins depends on the research approach adopted. For example, in some approaches, all of the data are collected before analysis begins. In others, such as grounded theory research, analysis occurs throughout the data collection, as data are constantly compared in order to build a theory.

Qualitative research can generate immense amounts of data, which the researcher needs to manage. Initially, the researcher needs to *immerse*

data immersion
the process by which the qualitative researcher absorbs themselves in data to extract content and meanings

coding
a process of marking keywords or phrases in text

themselves into the data to become familiar with their contents and meaning. **Data immersion** may require several readings of transcripts and multiple listenings to recordings. It is imperative that the researcher ensure the participants' intended meanings are not lost.

There are many ways to approach analysis of qualitative data. Most of these involve **coding** and then categorising data, which require a significant investment of time to do accurately. Coding involves working through each line or paragraph, depending on the overall approach, for data that address the research question. These segments of data are then marked, or coded. In the next step, codes are arranged into groups of similar meanings, where they can be further grouped into broad categories, which may have associated subcategories.

In some research approaches, there are specific processes for coding data. For example, in grounded theory there are different levels of coding: initial coding with early data collected; intermediate coding, known as *selective*, *axial* or *focused coding*, where categories and theory are emerging; and advanced coding, where there is finalising of the theory (Mills et al. 2014).

thematic analysis
an interpretive process of organising qualitative data into themes

inductive approach
an interpretive approach that seeks to develop a new theory or model from data, moving from specific observations to make generalisations

The two main approaches to data analysis reported in the nursing and midwifery research literature are *thematic analysis* and *content analysis*. Often, they are incorrectly interchanged, but they are different.

Thematic analysis

Thematic analysis involves taking an **inductive approach** to find meanings from data. There are many described approaches to undertaking thematic analysis. One common approach is described by Braun and Clarke (2006, p. 87) in a six-step process:

1   The researcher first familiarises themself with the data.
2   Next, initial codes are generated.
3   From the initial codes, the researcher searches to find patterns of similar ideas—that is, **themes**.

4   From this, the themes emerging from the dataset are reviewed and refined.

5   Next, each of the themes is defined and given a title or name.

6   Finally, the themes are reported.

Content analysis

There are various understandings as to what constitutes content analysis. It is considered more deductive in nature than thematic analysis, seeking to draw descriptive conclusions from the data, rather than broad understandings (Crowe et al. 2015). Content analysis is often suited to smaller qualitative datasets, such as those obtained through open-ended survey questions where there is insufficient data to create themes through thematic analysis.

> **theme**
> a grouping of data containing similar meanings; it emerges through thematic analysis

> **content analysis**
> a deductive process of analysing qualitative data; it can be done numerically or in categories

In some approaches to content analysis, qualitative data may be quantified. Polgar and Thomas (2013) describe such an approach whereby the meaningful pieces of text, particularly words or key terms, are counted and described in number format. They suggest that statistical analysis can then be applied to the data and hypotheses tested.

The researcher needs to determine whether they are going to approach data analysis manually, by labelling or highlighting text, or using computer-assisted qualitative data analysis, or CAQDAS. There are many software programs available to assist researchers, such as NVivo and ATLAS.ti. While still requiring the researcher to code data segments, these programs facilitate searching and grouping of data into patterns or categories.

In our case study, Jill undertakes ten semi-structured interviews. Each is audio-recorded and lasts between 48 and 56 minutes. She chooses to transcribe them herself, as she does not have the funding to send them to a professional transcriber. In total, she ends up with 300 pages of double-spaced text. In line with her theoretical approach, Jill chooses to use thematic analysis and finds two key themes emerging. Under each theme, there emerge sub-themes, as follows:

Theme 1: The nature of person-centred care in the ward
> Sub-theme: How person-centred care is being delivered
> Sub-theme: Factors impacting on person-centred care delivery

Theme 2: Staff readiness for person-centred care
> Sub-theme: Understandings of person-centred care and providing such care
> Sub-theme: Educational preparation of staff
> Sub-theme: Attitudes surrounding person-centred care

RESEARCH EXAMPLE 5.1 Using grounded theory to study woman-centred midwifery care

Barry et al. (2014) wanted to explore how new midwifery graduates apply midwifery philosophy of care in their first six months of practice. They chose grounded theory to underpin the study, as they wanted to examine the social processes graduates used. They interviewed eleven midwifery graduates as well as sourcing participant and interviewer journals to develop their theory. Data analysis led to the development of the substantive theory they called *transcending barriers*, which had three different stages; they labelled these *addressing personal attributes*, *understanding the bigger picture* and *evaluating, planning and acting*. Their findings assisted understanding of how new graduates begin to apply woman-centred care and provided information on how new midwives can be supported in their transition.

M.J. Barry, Y.L. Hauck, T. O'Donogue & S. Clarke, 2014, 'Newly-graduated midwives transcending barriers: Mechanisms for putting plans into action', *Midwifery*, vol. 30, pp. 962–967.

Questions for consideration

- Why was grounded theory an appropriate research approach for this study?
- How might the findings be used in midwifery education?

RESEARCH EXAMPLE 5.2 Using a qualitative descriptive approach to study person-centred care

Person-centred care is important for ensuring continuity of effective health care. A study by Rosengren (2016) used a qualitative descriptive approach to describe managers' experiences of implementation of person-centred care in Sweden. Person-centred care had been implemented; however, there was little known from managers' perspectives about its implementation. To explore this issue, Rosengren conducted individual interviews with eight first-line managers within the medical department who had more than one year of management experience and person-centred care. Interviews commenced with the question If I say *person-centred care*, what comes to mind? Responses led to subsequent questions. Interviews lasted between 42 and 63 minutes. Data were analysed using qualitative content analysis. From the analysis, three categories emerged that described their experiences: *structured approach—to be organised, care planning—to be continued* and *teamwork—to be together*. The findings were considered important in ensuring person-centred care is effectively implemented and ultimately improves healthcare provision.

K. Rosengren, 2016, 'Person-centred care: A qualitative study on first line managers' experiences on its implementation', *Health Services Management Research*, vol. 29, no. 3, pp. 42–49.

Questions for consideration

- Why was a descriptive qualitative research approach appropriate for this study?
- How might the findings be applied to nursing practice?

Ensuring quality of qualitative research

Qualitative research has been criticised as not being rigorous in its approaches. While that may be true of some qualitative research, there are, as with quantitative research, methods that researchers should employ to enhance the accuracy of the conclusions they draw. Key concepts include: *data saturation, credibility, fittingness (transferability), dependability, triangulation* and *confirmability*. In addition to these concepts, it is vital that qualitative researchers ensure that their research approach and design are consistent with their overarching philosophical approach. This means that their research question, sampling, data collection methods, data analysis and reporting should all be in line with the chosen approach.

Credibility

credibility
ensuring interpretations and conclusions drawn from data are truly reflective

member checking
the process of returning to participants to check interpretations made

Credibility is achieved when the interpretations and conclusions drawn by the researcher are truly reflective of the views and details presented by the participants. **Member checking** is one way in which credibility can be assessed: Using this, the researcher returns to participants to check that the interpretations represent their experiences accurately. This process can be undertaken verbally or by providing a written summary to participants (Cope 2014).

Fittingness

Fittingness, also known as **transferability**, is the degree to which research findings can be transferred and have similar meanings, to other, similar populations (Cope 2014). The researcher cannot measure this; rather, only users of the research can do so (Lincoln & Guba 1985). In reporting on fittingness, researchers generally recognise that their findings are not generalisable but may have meaning or resonance with others in similar situations.

fittingness or **transferability**
the capacity for conclusions from qualitative research to have similar meanings in other, similar populations

Dependability

Dependability is the consistency of findings in other, similar conditions. **Triangulation** is one way to promote research dependability, through the use of multiple methods or data sources that the researcher can verify and from which they can draw accurate conclusions. Carter et al. (2014) drew on previous work of Denzin (1978) to describe four types of triangulation that may be used to ensure the dependability of qualitative research:

1   **Method triangulation** A combination of data collection methods is used (such as interviews, observations, field notes and journaling) within one study.

2 **Investigator triangulation** More than one researcher undertakes the interpretation of data and drawing of conclusions.

3 **Theory triangulation** More than one theory is employed in analysing and interpreting data, assisting with supporting the conclusions drawn.

4 **Data source triangulation** Data are drawn from a range of sources (such as different types of participants) to ensure that multiple perspectives are captured.

> **dependability**
> the consistency of qualitative findings in other, similar conditions

> **triangulation**
> the use of multiple methods or data sources that the researcher can verify and from which they can draw accurate conclusions

Previously in this chapter, we discussed the concept of data saturation—that is, the point at which no new data are emerging. Achieving data saturation is particularly important for ensuring that data are complete and that key aspects of a phenomenon have not been left out of the final interpretations.

Confirmability

Confirmability refers to the degree to which the findings represent the participants' responses and viewpoints. In order to achieve confirmability, reporting of findings should use rich verbatim text quotes from participants that reinforce conclusions drawn (Cope 2014). Documentation of the research process is also an important consideration with regard to confirmability. Throughout the research process, researchers should maintain an audit trail, documenting the steps taken and decisions made, that could be followed by another researcher (Streubert & Carpenter 2011).

> **confirmability**
> the degree to which qualitative findings represent participants' perspectives

Reporting findings

While there is no specific approach to reporting qualitative findings, it is important to consider who the intended audience is and to write with them in mind, and to ensure the theoretical framework is in line with the employed methodology throughout. There are numerous elements that need to be included in the research report:

- **Background** Introduction to the study and what was already known about the topic.
- **Paradigm and theoretical framework** The philosophy underpinning the study.
- **Research problem, research aim and research question** The problem that the research is exploring, what the research aims to do, and the question guiding the study.
- **Method** Details of the method chosen—for example, if interviews were employed, the interview schedule, the number conducted, their setting and duration, how they were recorded and transcribed; if observations were employed, where they were conducted, the number conducted, the types of data collected.
- **Participants** Details about participants and how they were recruited into the study.
- **Ethical considerations** Steps taken to manage potential ethical issues, and details of approval by Human Research Ethics Committee.
- **Data analysis** Outline of selected approach and step-by-step description of how analysis was performed.

ACTIVITY 5.5 Analysing a qualitative research report

1 Search for a qualitative research paper on a topic that is of interest to you.
2 Carefully review the methods section. Note the strategies used by the researcher to ensure the quality of their findings.
3 Examine the way in which the research is reported through the paper.

Questions for consideration

- Were the quality-control strategies sufficiently rigorous?
- Were there other strategies that could have been employed to enhance their rigour?
- Does the paper clearly describe the necessary details of the research?
- Are there any research components missing from the paper?
- What are the strengths of the report?

- **Trustworthiness and rigour** Details of processes by which these were managed in regard to findings, with reference to credibility, transferability, dependability, confirmability and data saturation.
- **Findings** Presented as themes or categories, which may also contain sub-themes or subcategories; all conclusions evidenced through inclusion of appropriate participant quotations that clearly support each claim made; reflect views from a range of participants.

CHAPTER SUMMARY

Qualitative research is commonly performed in nursing and midwifery. It reflects the nature of human experience with which nurses and midwives continually engage and has many differences to quantitative approaches. There are various ways to do qualitative research, depending on the research aim and question. In this chapter, we have explored common qualitative approaches used in nursing and midwifery research, though many others can be utilised. Varied types of data can be used in qualitative research and can be analysed using methods such as thematic and content analysis, while rigour and trustworthiness can be achieved through a range of strategies.

CHAPTER REVIEW QUESTIONS

- What is meant by *qualitative research*?
- What are some of the common qualitative approaches used in nursing and midwifery research? How do they differ?
- What types of data do qualitative researchers collect?
- What are the main processes for qualitative data analysis?
- How is rigour achieved in qualitative research?

QUESTIONS FOR DISCUSSION

- What are some possible applications for qualitative research to nursing and/ or midwifery practice?
- How can nurses and midwives contribute to qualitative research knowledge and use?

- What are some of the challenges that might be faced in undertaking qualitative research?
- What strategies could be used to promote qualitative research in nursing and midwifery practice?

QUESTIONS FOR PERSONAL REFLECTION

- How could qualitative research be employed to improve nursing or midwifery care?
- What have you learnt about qualitative research while working through this chapter?

USEFUL WEB RESOURCES

Association for Qualitative Research <www.aqr.org.uk>

REFERENCES AND FURTHER READING

Adamson, E., Pow, J., Houston, F. & Redpath, P., 2016, 'Exploring the experiences of patients attending day hospitals in the rural Scotland: Capturing the patient's voice', *Journal of Clinical Nursing*, vol. 26, pp. 3044–3055.

Atchan, M., Davis, D. & Foureur, M., 2016, 'A methodological review of qualitative case study methodology in midwifery research', *Journal of Advanced Nursing*, vol. 72, no. 10, pp. 2259–2271.

Barry, M.J., Hauck, Y.L., O'Donogue, T., Clarke, S., 2014, 'Newly-graduated midwives transcending barriers: Mechanisms for putting plans into action', *Midwifery*, vol. 30, pp. 962–967.

Beardsmore, E. & McSherry, R., 2017, 'Healthcare workers' perceptions of organisation culture and the impact on the delivery of compassionate quality care', *Journal of Research in Nursing*, vol. 22, nos 1–2, pp. 42–56.

Braun, V. & Clarke, V., 2006, 'Using thematic analysis in psychology', *Qualitative Research in Psychology*, vol. 3, no. 2, pp. 77–101.

Carter, N., Bryant-Lukosius, D., DiCenso, A., Blythe, J. & Neville, A.J., 2014, 'The use of triangulation in qualitative research', *Oncology Nursing Forum*, vol. 41, no. 5, pp. 545–547.

Clissett, P., Porock, D., Harwood, R.H. & Gladman, J.R.F., 2013, 'The challenges of achieving person-centred care in acute hospitals: A qualitative study of people with dementia and their families', *International Journal of Nursing Studies*, vol. 50, pp. 1495–1503.

Cope, D.G., 2014, 'Methods and meanings: Credibility and trustworthiness of qualitative research', *Oncology Nursing Forum*, vol. 41, no. 1, pp. 89–91.

Coyne, E., Grafton, E. & Reid, A., 2016, 'Strategies to successfully recruit and engage clinical nurses as participants in qualitative clinical research', *Contemporary Nurse*, vol. 52, no. 6, pp. 669–676.

Crowe, M., Inder, M. & Porter, R., 2015, 'Conducting qualitative research in mental health: Thematic and content analyses', *Australian and New Zealand Journal of Psychiatry*, vol. 49, no. 7, pp. 616–623.

Denzin, N.K., 1978, *The Research Act: A theoretical introduction to sociological methods*, 2nd edn, New York: McGraw-Hill.

Florczak, K.L., 2017, 'Adding to the truth of the matter: The case for qualitative research', *Nursing Science Quarterly*, vol. 30, no. 4, pp. 296–299.

Flynn, M., Watmough, S., Wright, A. & Fry, K., 2010, 'Health research in context: Defining the research question and designing the study', *British Journal of Cardiac Nursing*, vol. 5, no. 7, pp. 346–349.

Fusch, P.I. & Ness, L.R., 2015, 'Are we there yet? Data saturation in qualitative research', *The Qualitative Report*, vol. 20, no. 9, pp. 1408–1416.

Hall, H., Griffiths, D. & McKenna, L., 2013, 'From Darwin to constructivism: The evolution of grounded theory', *Nurse Researcher*, vol. 20, no. 3, pp. 17–21.

Houghton, C., Casey, D. & Smyth, S., 2017, 'Selection, collection and analysis as sources of evidence in case study research', *Nurse Researcher*, vol. 24, no. 4, pp. 36–41.

Lewis, L.F., 2015, 'Putting "quality" in qualitative research: A guide to grounded theory for mental health nurses', *Journal of Psychiatric and Mental Health Nursing*, vol. 22, pp. 821–828.

Lincoln, Y.S. & Guba, E., 1985, *Naturalistic Inquiry*, Beverly Hills, CA: Sage.

Liquirish, S. & Siebold, C., 2011, 'Applying a contemporary grounded theory methodology', *Nurse Researcher*, vol. 18, no. 4, pp. 11–16.

Matua, G.A., 2015, 'Choosing phenomenology as a guiding principle for nursing research', *Nurse Researcher*, vol. 22, no. 4, pp. 30–34.

Miles, M., Francis, K., Chapman, Y. & Taylor, B., 2013, 'Exploring Heideggerian hermeneutic phenomenology: A perfect fit for midwifery research', *Women and Birth*, vol. 26, pp. 273–276.

Miles, M., Francis, K., Chapman, Y. & Taylor, B., 2013, 'Hermeneutic phenomenology: A methodology of choice for midwives', *International Journal of Nursing Practice*, vol. 19, pp. 409–414.

Mills, J. & Birks, M., 2014, *Qualitative Methodology: A practical guide*, London: Sage.

Mills, J., Birks, M. & Hoare, K., 2014, 'Grounded theory', in J. Mills & M. Birks (eds), *Qualitative Methodology: A practical guide*, London: Sage, pp. 107–121.

Polgar, S. & Thomas, S., 2013, *Introduction to Research in the Health Sciences*, Edinburgh: Churchill Livingstone Elsevier.

Rosengren, K., 2016, 'Person-centred care: A qualitative study on first line managers' experiences on its implementation', *Health Services Management Research*, vol. 29, no. 3, pp. 42–49.

Ryan, G.S., 2017, 'An introduction to the origins, history and principles of ethnography', *Nurse Researcher*, vol. 24, no. 4, pp. 15–21.

Streubert, H.J. & Carpenter, D.R., 2011, *Qualitative Research in Nursing: Advancing the humanistic imperative*, Philadelphia, PA: Wolters Kluwer.

Thelin, I.L., Lundgren, I. & Hermansson, E., 2014, 'Midwives' lived experience of caring during childbirth: A phenomenological study', *Sexual & Reproductive Healthcare*, vol. 5, pp. 113–118.

Wang, C. & Burris, M.A., 1997, 'Photovoice: Concept, methodology, and use for participatory needs assessment', *Health Education & Behavior*, vol. 24, no. 3, pp. 369–387.

Wolf, A., 2017, 'What qualitative research can do for you: Deriving solutions and interventions from qualitative findings', *Journal of Emergency Nursing*, vol. 43, no. 5, pp. 484–485.

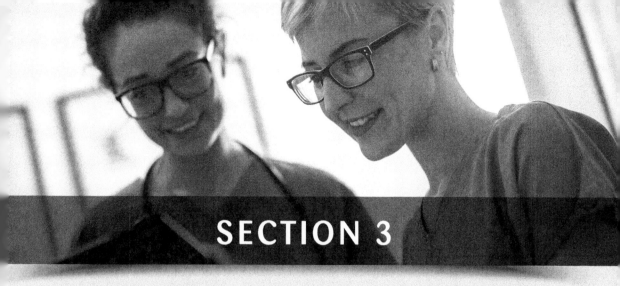

SECTION 3

HOW DO I CRITICALLY EVALUATE RESEARCH STUDIES?

Critique involves a detailed process of evaluation of research. It is paramount for nurses and midwives to ensure that the best possible evidence is being used in practice. The implementation of substandard or poorly designed research outcomes could lead to poor and inappropriate care delivery and have detrimental outcomes for those being cared for. This section centres on how to approach critical research reviews.

Chapter 6 focuses on the steps involved in making judgements about the quality of published research. It begins by looking at how to approach critiquing an individual research report. The second part of the chapter presents two increasingly popular types of critical literature reviews—namely, the scoping review and the systematic review, which involve analysing a group of research studies on a topic.

Chapter 7 focuses on ethical considerations in human research. Understanding these is crucial to being able to fully critique practical aspects of research approaches. It involves how ethical principles apply to research, as well as the roles of Human Research Ethics Committees and researchers with regard to the ethical conduct of research.

CHAPTER 6

Critiquing research

LEARNING OBJECTIVES

After working through this chapter, you should be able to:

- discuss what is meant by *critique* of a research study
- outline the steps involved in undertaking a critique of research
- discuss ways in which author and journal quality can be evaluated
- discuss the roles of systematic and scoping reviews in research critique
- explain the differences between systematic and scoping reviews.

KEY TERMS AND CONCEPTS

Critique, H-index, impact factor, journal quality, predatory journals, quartile ranking, research quality, scoping review, systematic review

CASE STUDY OVERVIEW

Alice is a clinical nurse specialist who is interested in the effectiveness of vital signs monitoring in her ward. She suspects that nurses on the ward are missing key changes in patients' conditions. Knowing that subtle changes can indicate early deterioration in a patient's status, she is concerned that early changes in vital signs are not being detected and deterioration is only being identified when it is well established.

CHAPTER INTRODUCTION

Over the past decade, the volume of available research to inform nursing and midwifery practice has exploded and continues to grow every day. This makes it difficult to keep up-to-date with evidence to support best clinical practice. Unfortunately, the quality of the available research can vary significantly, so the ability to critique it becomes very important. In this chapter, we will work through the process of critiquing research studies. In the second half of the chapter, we will explore some structured review approaches to critiquing bodies of research that are becoming popular in nursing and midwifery—namely, the systematic review and scoping review—as means of managing the large body of research that exists in any one topic area.

Critiquing and evaluating research quality

The ability to **critique** research is important for students at both under-graduate and postgraduate levels. Qualified nurses and midwives also need this ability, as they may be invited to provide peer-reviewed critique of research submitted for consideration for publication in journals. Furthermore, healthcare professionals need to be able to effectively critique research studies to ensure that they are delivering best practice to the people they care for and that they are not implementing practice interventions based on poorly designed research. Many people incorrectly think of *critique* as criticising or finding faults in a work. While this may happen in the process, proper critique involves taking an objective view in assessing a research study to identify its strengths and weaknesses and how the findings apply to practice.

critique
assessment of a research study to identify strengths, weaknesses and quality

Effective critique of research is appropriately complex. Regardless of whether you are reviewing papers for an assignment or a literature review, there are some key steps in critiquing and evaluating the quality of published research studies.

Title

The title should clearly indicate what the paper is about and should be short. Often, journals limit the number of words contained in titles, by requiring them to be no more than ten words long, for example. In many journals, the type of research study being reported on is also included in the title. Questions to ask of the title include:

- Does it indicate what the paper is about?
- Does it reflect the research undertaken?
- Is it clear and appropriately written?

Author

Details about the author (or authors) are essential considerations. It is important to assess whether the researcher (or researchers) is affiliated with a reputable institution, such as a hospital or university. In addition, where possible, it is good to explore whether they have a qualification in which they have learnt research skills, such as a masters by research or doctor of philosophy (PhD). One measure of a researcher's output is the **H-index**, which measures the number of citations received by a researcher, according to their most-cited articles. For example, a researcher who has been cited ten or more times in ten publications has an H-index of 10. The higher the H-index, the better. In nursing and midwifery, H-indexes are relatively low compared to other fields. McKenna et al. (2017) analysed the research publication performance of Australian nursing and midwifery professors and found the median H-index was 14 for professors and 7 for associate professors. Questions to consider about the author include:

H-index
a measure of a researcher's publication citations

- Are they affiliated with a reputable institution?
- Do they have research qualifications?
- What is their H-index?

Journal

There is great diversity in the quality of journals themselves. Evaluating them is complex but important in assessing the overall quality of the research being published. It is likely that better journals publish better quality research papers. There are many bogus journals, known as **predatory journals**, which appear legitimate and reputable but are anything but. Often, these so-called journals do not have appropriate peer review (review by peers in the relevant field) processes in place for reviewing manuscripts and no editorial boards to monitor journal quality; they exist merely to make money out of inexperienced researchers.

predatory journal
a non-credible journal that exploits researchers by charging publication fees without providing academic oversight and rigour, such as peer review

They often publish one or two volumes then disappear with the work of a researcher whose own long-term credibility is threatened by publishing with them (Darbyshire et al. 2017; Oermann et al. 2016). Predatory publishers may publish work that credible journals would not and that may be based on flawed research processes. The ability to critique journal quality is, therefore, paramount to ensuring that only high-quality research is being implemented into clinical practice.

Journal quality can be assessed in a variety of ways. First, the journal should have a credible editor in charge. Therefore, it is worth finding out a bit about the editor, which can be done easily. They should be supported by an editorial board, associate editors or both. Second, the journal should have a sound, documented process for managing peer review of manuscripts. Umlauf (2016) suggests that promise of rapid review and publication should be a red flag for authors, as quality reviews take some time to complete. Third, the journal should be published by a credible organisation—usually a recognised publisher or a professional institution. Journals that are sound will be members of the Committee on Publication Ethics (or COPE) and in the case of nursing and midwifery should also be on the International Academy of Nursing Editors (or INANE) journal listing.

The best of the credible journals can be determined using additional strategies to rank them on a range of criteria; the two most commonly

quartile ranking
ranking of journals into four categories, where the 1st quartile, or top 25 per cent (Q1), contains the highest-ranking journals

used are quartile ranking and impact factor. **Quartile ranking** orders all of the journals in a discipline according to quality criteria and then groups them into the top 25 per cent (Q1), second 25 per cent (Q2), third 25 per cent (Q3) and bottom 25 per cent (Q4). The best journals, therefore, are those in Q1, which constitutes the top 25 per cent for that field. The SCImago Journal & Country Rank (or SJR) indicator takes this approach and is easily accessible. The **impact factor** measures the average citations of papers from a particular journal. For example, if a journal has an impact factor of 1.35, this indicates that on average each paper published in that journal is cited by other papers 1.35 times. The higher the impact

impact factor
a measure of the impact of a journal, relating to citations of the papers that it publishes

factor, the higher the impact and quality of the journal. Again, in nursing and midwifery, impact factors are lower than in other disciplines. In 2017, nursing impact factors ranged from 3.656 (for the *International Journal of Nursing Studies*) to 0.404. It is important to note that not all credible journals have an impact factor, as it can take many years to qualify. Impact factor information can be sourced in various places, such as journal websites; at the International Scientific Institute's Journal Impact Factor List (see Research tip 6.1); and through databases accessible through your library, such as Scopus and Web of Science. As will be clear now, evaluating the quality of a journal is complex but important in assessing the overall quality of the research being published. Questions to ask of a journal include:

- Is it a reputable journal?
- What types of papers does it publish?
- Does it have a recognised editor and editorial board?
- Is it published on listings of credible journals?
- What is its quartile ranking?
- What is its impact factor (if applicable)?

RESEARCH TIP 6.1 Places to check for journal credibility

- Databases like Scopus or Web of Science, which should be accessible through your institution's library
- Directory of Open Access Journals <https://doaj.org>
- International Academy of Nursing Editors' Directory of Nursing Journals <https://nursingeditors.com/journals-directory/>
- International Scientific Institute's Journal Impact Factor List <www.scijournal.org>
- SCImago Journal & Country Rank <www.scimagojr.com>

Abstract

The abstract is a short summary of the paper, around 100 to 300 words in length depending on the journal. From it, you should get a sense of the whole study. It should provide an overview of the background to the study; the aim or problem being researched; the research design, data collection and data analysis approaches; key findings; and recommendations or implications for practice. Questions to ask of the abstract include:

- Does it provide an overview of how the whole study was conducted?
- Does it provide recommendations or implications for practice?

Introduction and background literature review

This section tells you a lot about the planning undertaken for the research and the current knowledge in the field being researched. It should be focused and demonstrate the deficits or gaps in existing research, justifying why the current study is needed. Questions to ask about the introduction and background literature review include:

- Do they demonstrate a sound understanding and overview of the topic and what is already known?
- Are all the key previous studies mentioned?
- Are the sources used original, that is, primary sources?
- Is information taken from other studies used out of its original context?
- Is there critical review of the literature?
- Does the review demonstrate a gap in existing knowledge?
- Is the problem clearly identified?

Methodology

The methodology presents the theoretical framework underpinning the research study. In qualitative studies, this may include an overview of a philosophical position, such as phenomenology or grounded theory. It presents the lens through which the study was conducted, such as how the data were collected and analysed. Questions to ask of the methodology include:

- Is the aim of the study clearly stated?
- Is the theoretical approach consistent with the study aim?
- For qualitative studies, is the underlying philosophical position described?

Study design

The study design should align directly with the chosen methodology and the research aim or question and the data collection methods should be described. The section should demonstrate how rigour was achieved in the research process. Research tools should be described in detail. How this is done depends largely on the type of study being reported. For example, if a questionnaire was used, it would be important to understand how it was developed and validated and, if it was a new tool, piloted. If qualitative interviews were used, the interview guide should be presented, listing the key interview questions and highlighting how the research aim or question was being addressed. In addition, the study participants should be described in detail including how they were selected for inclusion in the study, how they were recruited to the study and what their participation entailed. Questions to ask about the study design include:

- Is the research design consistent with the research aim?
- Is the design clearly explained and recognisable?
- Are participants well described?
- Who was included and who was excluded?
- How were participants sampled and recruited?
- Is the sample size sufficient to draw meaningful conclusions?
- Are the research instruments appropriate to answer the research question?
- Are these instruments valid and reliable?
- Was a pilot study conducted?

Ethical considerations

Ethical considerations with regard to research on humans are covered in detail in Chapter 7. Any research that involves humans must adhere to strict guidelines and processes to ensure that the rights and safety of the person are upheld throughout. All researchers engaging in research are expected to describe the steps taken to ensure that these are managed appropriately. Questions that need to be posed with regard to this aspect include:

- Are relevant ethical considerations discussed?
- Were potential ethical issues appropriately managed?
- Is there a statement indicating that the study was approved by a Human Research Ethics Committee?

Data collection

Each of the data collection methods used in the study needs to be fully described. If using questionnaires, researchers need to describe how these were developed, how they were distributed and managed. If using interviews, the questions guiding the interviews should be presented. The time at which data were collected is also important; if data are old, findings may be irrelevant to current practice. Furthermore, the setting in which the data were collected may not be applicable to local practice settings, so implementation in other places may not be appropriate. Questions to ask about data collection include:

- When and where were the data collected?
- Were the data collection methods appropriate for the chosen methodology and research question?
- If appropriate, how were participants assigned to groups?
- Are the data collection methods justified by the authors?

Data analysis

In this section, the processes by which data were managed and analysed need to be fully explained. For statistical data, the tests conducted on them should be outlined, and these tests need to be clearly appropriate for types of data obtained. For qualitative data, how they were coded and grouped also requires clear description. Questions to ask about data analysis include:

- Are the processes by which the data were analysed fully explained?
- Were these processes appropriate for the chosen methodology and research design?
- For quantitative research, were the appropriate statistical tests performed? Were they accurate? Are they appropriately presented?
- For qualitative research, is the way in which data were managed well explained?
- Is the presentation of findings consistent with the chosen methodology?
- How were findings verified?

Interpretation of results

Interpretation of results is usually included in the discussion section of the research report. The findings of the study are positioned in the context of what is already known about the topic, showing how the new findings contribute to the existing body of knowledge. Issues arising or limitations in the study need to be fully and clearly described, and there should be recommendations for future research, practice or education. Questions to ask about the interpretation of results include:

- Did the study answer the research question or aim?
- Are the researcher's conclusions supported by the findings?
- Are the findings generalisable? If not, are they representative of the broader population?
- Has any potential bias been identified?
- Are the limitations of the study explained? Are they sufficient?
- Are implications and recommendations for practice or future research presented?
- What new questions have emerged?
- Is the new knowledge generated made explicit?

Conflicts of interest

Research should be free of any potential bias. It is important to examine whether there are potential areas where the researchers may have experienced conflicts of interest. Funding is one area where this may arise, as well as any vested interest in a study, such as if a drug or device is being tested that might later be profitable. Questions to ask about conflicts of interest include:

- Was the study externally funded? If so, by whom?
- Are there any potential conflicts of interest?

ACTIVITY 6.1 Undertaking a research report critique

1 Search one of your library's databases for a study related to vital signs monitoring in nursing or midwifery, or another topic of personal interest.
2 Work through each of the steps described in this chapter for critiquing published research.
3 Summarise your key conclusions.

RESEARCH EXAMPLE 6.1 Observation of nurses' practices in monitoring vital signs

Early recognition of patient deterioration can reduce the risk of potential harm. Timeliness and accuracy of vital signs monitoring can be key to early recognition. Cardona-Morrell et al. (2016) sought to explore nurses' vital signs monitoring practices on a medical ward and an acute surgical ward in New South Wales, Australia. They employed direct observation of nurses in practice, along with patient interactions. In total, they observed 441 patient interactions by 42 nurses. The five minimum vital signs measurements required by local policy were only performed in 6–21 per cent of occasions. Furthermore, measurements were only documented immediately in 93 per cent of cases, and nurse–patient interactions only occurred in 88 per cent of observations.

M. Cardona-Morrell, M. Prgomet, R. Lake, M. Nicholson, R. Harrison, J. Long, J. Westbrook, J. Braithwaite & K. Hillman, 2016, 'Vital signs monitoring and nurse–patient interaction: A qualitative observational study of hospital practice', *International Journal of Nursing Studies*, vol. 56, pp. 9–16.

Questions for consideration

- What issues might arise from an observational study like this?
- How might the findings from this study be used to support improved practice?

RESEARCH EXAMPLE 6.2 A survey to assess nursing students' monitoring of vital signs

---

Recognition of early deterioration is an important role for nurses. Leonard and Kyriacos (2015) conducted a study with final-year undergraduate nursing students to explore whether they could recognise abnormal physiological vital signs measurements in order to seek assistance to manage deteriorating patients. The researchers used an adapted survey that covered seven physiological variables: temperature, respiratory rate, heart rate, systolic blood pressure, urinary output, oxygen saturation and level of consciousness. Findings suggested that students recognised normal temperature readings but otherwise had difficulty identifying early signs of deterioration. This indicated that they would delay seeking skilled assistance until patients' conditions were at a critical level.

M. Leonard & U. Kyriacos, 2015, 'Student nurses' recognition of early signs of abnormal vital sign recording', *Nurse Education Today*, vol. 35, pp. e11–e18.

Questions for consideration

- How might the findings from this study inform the delivery of undergraduate education?
- What might the long-term implications of this study be for patients?

Critiquing tools

There are several tools available to assist users of research, as well as researchers, with quality reviews of research studies and working through the increasing amount of research generated. The EQUATOR (Enhancing the Quality and Transparency of Health Research) Network serves as a repository for many critical appraisal tools which have been validated as checklists for different types of research. Examples of these are presented in Research tip 6.2. In addition, the Joanna Briggs Institute (2017) and the Critical Appraisal Skills Programme (2018; or CASP), have developed suites of critical appraisal tools for a vast array of study designs.

RESEARCH TIP 6.2 Examples of study reporting guidelines

AGREE	Clinical practice guidelines
CARE	Case reports
CONSORT	Randomised controlled trials
PRISMA	Systematic reviews
SQUIRE	Quality improvement studies
SRQR	Qualitative research
STROBE	Observational studies

All are accessible through the EQUATOR Network, at <www.equator-network.org>.

ACTIVITY 6.2 Using critical appraisal tools

1 Using the research article you sourced in Activity 6.1, go to the EQUATOR Network website, at <www.equator-network.org>, the Joanna Briggs Institute (2017) website and the Critical Appraisal Skills Programme (2018) website and source the appropriate reporting guidelines for the study.
2 Use the reporting guidelines to undertake an evaluation of the quality of the research. Note down your conclusions.

Questions for consideration
- How do your conclusions compare with the review you conducted in Activity 6.1?
- How useful did you find the critical appraisal tools?

Structured critical literature review

In the previous part of this chapter, we explored critiquing individual research studies in detail, as well as using critical appraisal tools. In this section, we will look at approaches to performing structured critical reviews of a body of similar work. This is an important practice, as conclusions drawn from such reviews can ensure that the best evidence is applied to nursing and midwifery practice.

Previously, it was acceptable to perform **traditional narrative reviews** of literature. These have no particular approach or structure, are subjective in nature and are often based upon the author's selective approach. Hence, they can be heavily biased and unsystematic (Aromataris & Pearson 2014), lack critical appraisal and fail to include the best available research studies. It could be detrimental to base nursing or midwifery practice on the findings of such reviews. Hence, there is a need for very structured, protocol-driven approaches to examining and synthesising the vast amount of literature that may exist on a particular topic in order to extract the best evidence to inform the delivery of care. Among the most common structured critical literature reviews used in nursing and midwifery are the *systematic review* and the *scoping review*, which we will examine below.

> **traditional narrative review**
> a subjective, non-critical review of the literature where included research is selected by the author

Systematic review

In this section, we will build on the concept of the **systematic review** introduced in Chapter 1. As its title implies, this type of review is conducted in a systematic way. Aromataris and Pearson (2014, p. 54) identify key characteristics of a systematic review and the way in which is it conducted, stating that it has:

> **systematic review**
> a literature review that uses a structured question and search approach, along with critical appraisal and quality analysis of studies

- clearly articulated objectives and questions to be addressed
- inclusion and exclusion criteria, stipulated in the review protocol or proposal, that determine the eligibility of studies
- a comprehensive search to identify all relevant studies, both published and unpublished
- quality appraisal of included studies, assessment of the validity of their results and reporting of any exclusions based on quality
- analysis of data extracted from the included research
- presentation and synthesis of the findings extracted
- clear and transparent recording of the methodology and methods to conduct the review.

Systematic reviews provide high-level evidence that can be applied to practice through the synthesis of multiple studies. This synthesis adds strength that may not be achieved through a sole study.

1   Developing a review question and PICO

PICO
an acronym used to name the key aspects of a systematic review, usually referring to *population, intervention, comparator* and *outcome*

The first step in conducting a systematic review involves developing the research question. This should be carefully thought through, as it needs to be searchable and answerable. It also must incorporate a PICO statement. *PICO* is an acronym used to define the key aspects of a systematic review:

- **P**opulation The types of participants who will be the focus of the review
- **I**ntervention The intervention or phenomenon of interest that is being examined
- **C**omparator What the intervention or phenomenon of interest is being compared with
- **O**utcome The outcome measures that are being studied.

There are some variations on the PICO acronym. For systematic reviews of qualitative studies, PICO refers to the following:

- **P**opulation The types of participants who will be the focus of the review
- Phenomenon of **i**nterest The concept being studied
- **Co**ntext The setting in which the study should be situated.

Others use *PICOT*, where the *T* refers to a *timeframe*; or *PICOS*, where the *S* refers to *study designs*.

In this chapter's case study, we could pose the review question *What is the effect of respiratory-rate monitoring in early detection of patient deterioration?* For this, our PICO would be:

- **P**opulation   Deteriorating patients
- **I**ntervention   Respiratory-rate monitoring
- **C**omparator   No respiratory rate monitoring
- **O**utcome   Early detection of deterioration.

2 *Developing the review protocol*

Once the question and PICO have been determined, the next step involves developing the **review protocol**, which will direct the search for relevant articles and how these will be analysed and reported. A key part of the protocol involves defining the review's inclusion criteria, which decide whether a study will be included or not and might involve such things as the languages that studies are written in, the timeframe in which research was published, specific characteristics of participants (such as age range or gender), databases and other sources to be searched and the types of studies. The protocol should also identify the quality appraisal tools to be used and how the data will be extracted and analysed.

review protocol
a detailed plan for undertaking a systematic or scoping review

The review protocol will also include the key search terms (keywords). As we saw in Chapter 2, these can be difficult to determine, need to be constructed in such a way that they will find relevant articles and may vary between databases. Usually, a preliminary list of keywords is developed, followed by detailed development of search strings for each database to be used (see Aromataris and Riitano 2014; US National Library of Medicine 2018). Librarians are highly skilled in formulating search strategies, so seeking their assistance with the formulation of key search terms is advisable. Using our case study, we might develop our protocol in the following way:

- **Inclusion criteria** Quantitative studies published between 2007 and 2017 in English
- **Search strategy**
  - Databases MEDLINE, CINAHL, PubMed
  - Grey literature Google Scholar, professional organisation websites
  - Handsearching Reference lists of retrieved studies
  - Initial key search terms *Patient AND deteriorat* AND nurse AND respiratory rate AND monitor* OR measur* AND detect* AND early OR missed OR late*
- **Quality appraisal** Critical Appraisal Skills Programme checklists appropriate to the studies.

Note the way in which the key terms are shortened when there might be different forms of the same stem word, such as *deteriorate*, *deteriorating* and *deterioration*. By using a truncator symbol (in this case an asterisk), we can find all of these and not miss relevant papers. Note also the reference to *grey literature*: other relevant studies that might not be listed in databases but might be available from other places—for example, websites of professional or government organisations. You might even use *handsearching*, by looking at reference lists of research studies located in the search to find other studies that may have been missed.

3   *Conducting the search, selecting retrieved studies*

Once the review protocol has been sufficiently refined, the search is conducted. It is important to keep accurate records of each step. From the initial search, it is common to source large numbers of papers. When numerous databases are being used, first, duplicate records are removed. Following this, the remaining titles and abstracts are read to determine if they fit the inclusion criteria, with those deemed not relevant removed. Ideally, this significantly reduces the number of records. Full texts of the reports that are left are then assessed for inclusion, and again some are

---

ACTIVITY 6.3 Developing a systematic review protocol

Think back to our case study of Alice who was interested in the effectiveness of vital signs monitoring for early detection of patient deterioration. Prior to doing research in her ward, Alice decides to undertake a systematic review of existing literature to explore the topic. She comes up with the following question to guide her systematic review: *How effective are vital signs measurements in detecting early patient deterioration?*

Draft a brief protocol that Alice could use to undertake a systematic review. Use the following headings:

Title
Review question
Background
Inclusion criteria

- Participants
- Phenomenon or intervention of interest
- Outcomes
- Study types

Search strategy

---

normally taken out. This leaves a much smaller number of studies for inclusion in the final review. Often, these steps are presented in a visual Preferred Reporting Items for Systematic Reviews and Meta-Analyses (or PRISMA) flow chart (see <http://prisma-statement.org>). In our case study, the flow chart might look like the one in Figure 6.1.

4 *Appraising retrieved studies, extracting and synthesising data*

The quality appraisal tools listed in the review protocol are used to assess the articles included so far. These enable assessment of the quality of the studies included in the final review. At this point, studies not meeting a particular level of quality are removed, and this further reduces the

FIGURE 6.1 Flow chart of a search

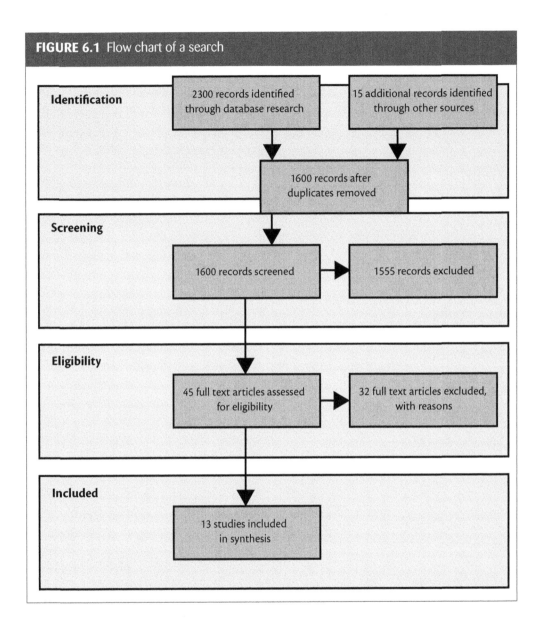

number of studies being included in the final review. According to Porritt et al. (2014), the process of quality appraisal involves establishing risk of bias (in selection, performance, detection and attrition) as well as external validity—how generalisable findings are and, as a result, how applicable they are to making practice changes.

Data extraction and synthesis methods vary; however, protocol development often leads to decisions over what data are important to extract. Usually, these data are presented in the form of tables, which are then interpreted. From this, conclusions can be drawn. At this point, Roberston-Malt (2014) suggests reporting on the implications for practice according to Joanna Briggs Institute recommendations regarding evidence of feasibility of implementation, appropriateness to the clinical situation, meaningfulness of the intervention for patients and effectiveness of the intervention.

data extraction
the process of selecting data from studies for inclusion in a systematic or scoping review

---

ACTIVITY 6.4 Exploring systematic reviews

Using your library's databases, conduct a search for systematic reviews on a topic of personal interest. Identify two or three to read and get a feel for how systematic reviews are reported and presented.

Questions for consideration

- What structure is used to present the findings?
- How are the reviews used to elicit key findings and recommendations that could be translated to practice?

RESEARCH EXAMPLE 6.3 A nursing systematic review

Failure to recognise early change in a patient's status may lead to unnecessary morbidity and mortality. Many healthcare settings have implemented early warning scoring systems to avoid these outcomes. However, Odell et al. (2009) believed that the effectiveness of these systems was not clear, so they undertook a systematic review to examine research relating to nursing observation practice and detection of deterioration in general ward patients. They searched four databases for relevant studies dating from 1990 to 2007. Fourteen studies met their inclusion and quality criteria. They performed their analysis by grouping findings into themes: *recognition, recording, reviewing* and *reporting*. They reported a complex and multifactorial process. Nurses used intuition in detecting deterioration, with vital signs being used to validate their feelings. Overall, the researchers concluded that there was insufficient research evidence of suitable quality in the area. Despite reports of implementation of detection and management systems for deterioration, they felt that timeliness and effective processes were needed to fully optimise the systems.

M. Odell, C. Victor & D. Oliver, 2009, 'Nurses' role in detecting deterioration in ward patients: Systematic literature review', *Journal of Advanced Nursing*, vol. 65, no. 10, pp. 1992–2006.

Questions for consideration

- How has the systematic review described above provided greater scope in understanding this issue?
- Why is the conclusion from this review more powerful, through combining the findings from a number of research studies, than looking at just one study?

Scoping review

The scoping review is a newer approach to undertaking a structured appraisal of a broad topic of interest and is becoming particularly popular in nursing and midwifery. It reportedly initially emerged in the social sciences, where structured systematic reviews were viewed as very narrow and prescriptive for the types of research conducted in those related disciplines (Thomas et al. 2017). Scoping reviews are applicable to nursing and midwifery, as they incorporate both science and social perspectives. Furthermore, where systematic reviews often focus on the effectiveness of an intervention, scoping reviews seek to expose the

scoping review
a structured literature review that employs a protocol to explore a broad topic area, sometimes to identify gaps in what is known

gaps in what is currently known about a topic (Thomas et al. 2017). This makes them of relevance to the identification of new research opportunities.

While many of the steps undertaken are in line with those of a systematic review, scoping reviews are performed a little differently. They still require the development of a protocol, but rather than using a PICO statement scoping reviews employ different frameworks. The Joanna Briggs Institute (2015) approach to scoping reviews suggests a framework encompassing *types of participants*, *concept* and *context*:

- **Types of participants** This section clearly identifies who the participants of interest are, along with their particular characteristics.
- **Concept** This is the topic being reviewed; it could be an intervention, phenomenon, construct or concept.
- **Context** The context is the specific setting which is being explored—for example, a clinical, community or educational setting.

Think back to our case study of Alice who was interested in the effectiveness of vital signs monitoring for early detection of patient deterioration. Alice decides she needs to undertake a scoping review to see what is known about nurses' routines in vital signs monitoring. She comes up with the following question to guide her scoping review: *What is known about nurses' routines in vital signs monitoring?* The question is much broader than it would be for a systematic review. For this, the inclusion criteria would be:

- **Types of participants** Nurses
- **Concept** Routines
- **Context** Vital signs monitoring.

ACTIVITY 6.5 Developing a scoping review protocol

In our case study, Alice finally decides she needs some more broad information and uses the following question to guide her review: *What is known about nurses' roles in detecting early patient deterioration?*

Draft a protocol for this review, using the following headings, which are informed by the Joanna Briggs Institute (2015) methodology for scoping reviews:

Title
Review question
Background
Inclusion criteria

- Types of participants
- Concept
- Context

Search strategy
Data extraction

ACTIVITY 6.6 Exploring scoping reviews

Using your library's databases, conduct a search for scoping reviews on a topic of personal interest. Identify two or three to read and get a feel for how scoping reviews are reported and presented.

Questions for consideration
- What are the key aspects that seem similar across the reviews?
- Are there differences in the ways in which each is presented?
- Are there differences between these scoping reviews and what you have found previously in systematic reviews?

RESEARCH EXAMPLE 6.4 A midwifery scoping review

Electronic fetal monitoring is an important monitoring role for midwives and is becoming routine in many places. Paterno et al. (2016) wanted to explore research on electronic fetal monitoring use and low-risk birthing women. They conducted a scoping review of published research from 1996 that examined caesarean section and electronic fetal monitoring use in this group of women. In the review, they screened 57 full text articles, of which seven were included in the final review. They concluded that the findings suggested an association between caesearean section and electronic fetal monitoring but recommended further studies be undertaken, along with other technologies that might increase caesarean section rates. They also suggested that future studies explore benefits and risks of electronic fetal monitoring versus fetal heart auscultation for low-risk women.

M.T. Paterno, K. McElroy & M. Regan, 2016, 'Electronic fetal monitoring and caesarean birth: A scoping review', *Birth*, vol. 43, no. 4, pp. 277–284.

Questions for consideration

- Why was a scoping review the most appropriate approach to addressing the researchers' questions?
- How is a scoping review different from a systematic review?

CHAPTER SUMMARY

Evidence to support nursing, midwifery and health professional practice more broadly is flourishing. Nurses and midwives need to possess skills to sift through the available evidence and effectively critique it for potential implementation into practice and the delivery of care. Without such capabilities, patient care may be compromised through implementation of inappropriate or poorly developed research evidence. This chapter has examined the processes for critiquing individual research studies and has introduced the systematic review and scoping review as means of critiquing bodies of research.

CHAPTER REVIEW QUESTIONS

- What is meant by *critique* of a research study?
- What are the key aspects to be reviewed in a critique?
- How can author and journal quality be evaluated?
- How are systematic and scoping reviews different?
- Why are systematic and scoping reviews particularly useful in nursing and midwifery?

QUESTIONS FOR DISCUSSION

- How does critiquing research papers challenge traditional narrative literature reviews?
- How might structured critical reviews enhance nursing and midwifery practice?
- What role do traditional narrative literature reviews play?

QUESTIONS FOR PERSONAL REFLECTION

- How has your learning from this chapter impacted on your perceptions of doing literature reviews?
- How might it change how you do these in future?
- How might you utilise scoping and systematic reviews in your practice?

USEFUL WEB RESOURCES

Cochrane <www.cochrane.org>

Critical Appraisal Skills Programme <www.casp-uk.net>

Directory of Open Access Journals <https://doaj.org>

Enhancing the Quality and Transparency of Health Research Network <www.equator-network.org>

International Academy of Nursing Editors' Directory of Nursing Journals <https://nursingeditors.com/journals-directory/>

International Scientific Institute's Journal Impact Factor List <www.scijournal.org>

Joanna Briggs Institute <http://joannabriggs.org>

Preferred Reporting Items for Systematic Reviews and Meta-Analyses <http://prisma-statement.org>

SCImago Journal & Country Rank <www.scimagojr.com>

REFERENCES AND FURTHER READING

Alderson, D., 2016, 'How to critically appraise a research paper', *Paediatrics and Child Health*, vol. 26, no. 3, pp. 110–113.

Aromataris, E. & Pearson, A., 2014, 'The systematic review: An overview', *American Journal of Nursing*, vol. 114, no. 3, pp. 53–58.

Aromataris, E. & Riitano, D., 2014, 'Constructing a search strategy and searching for evidence', *American Journal of Nursing*, vol. 114, no. 5, pp. 49–56.

Buccheri, R.K., 2017, 'Critical appraisal tools and reporting guidelines for evidence-based practice', *Worldviews of Evidence-Based Nursing*, vol. 14, no. 6, pp. 463–472.

Cardona-Morrell, M., Prgomet, M., Lake, R., Nicholson, M., Harrison, R., Long, J., Westbrook, J., Braithwaite, J. & Hillman, K., 2016, 'Vital signs monitoring and nurse–patient interaction: A qualitative observational study of hospital practice', *International Journal of Nursing Studies*, vol. 56, pp. 9–16.

Coughlin, S. & Molyneux, D., 2010, 'Consensus paper: Resources for teaching critical appraisal', *Education for Primary Care*, vol. 21, pp. 79–82.

Critical Appraisal Skills Programme, 2018, *CASP Checklists*, <https://casp-uk.net/casp-tools-checklists/>.

Darbyshire, P., McKenna, L., Lee, S.F. & East, C.E., 2017, 'Taking a stand against predatory publishers', *Journal of Advanced Nursing*, vol. 73, no. 7, pp. 1535–1537.

Davis, K., Drey, M. & Gould, D., 2009, 'What are scoping studies? A review of the nursing literature', *International Journal of Nursing Studies*, vol. 46, pp. 1386–1400.

Fawkes, C., Ward, E. & Carnes, D., 2015, 'What evidence is good evidence? A masterclass in critical appraisal', *International Journal of Osteopathic Medicine*, vol. 18, pp. 116–129.

Heywaert, M., Hannes, K., Maes, B. & Onghena, P., 2013, 'Critical appraisal of mixed methods studies', *Journal of Mixed Methods Research*, vol. 7, no. 4, pp. 302–327.

Joanna Briggs Institute, 2015, *The Joanna Briggs Institute Reviewers' Manual 2015: Methodology for JBI scoping reviews*, <http://joannabriggs.org/assets/docs/sumari/Reviewers-Manual_Methodology-for-JBI-Scoping-Reviews_2015_v2.pdf>.

Joanna Briggs Institute, 2017, *Critical Appraisal Tools*, <http://joannabriggs.org/research/critical-appraisal-tools.html>.

Leonard, M. & Kyriacos, U., 2015, 'Student nurses' recognition of early signs of abnormal vital sign recording', *Nurse Education Today*, vol. 35, pp. e11–e18.

McKenna, L., Cooper, S., Cant, R. & Bogossian, F., 2017, 'Research publication performance of Australian professors of nursing & midwifery', *Journal of Advanced Nursing*, doi: 10.1111/jan.13338.

Munn, Z., Tufanaru, C. & Aromataris, E., 2014, 'Data extraction and synthesis', *American Journal of Nursing*, vol. 114, no. 7, pp. 49–54.

Needleman, I., Clarkson, J. & Worthington, H., 2013, 'A practitioner's guide to developing critical appraisal skills', *Journal of the American Dental Association*, vol. 144, no. 5, pp. 527–530.

Odell, M., Victor, C. & Oliver, D., 2009, 'Nurses' role in detecting deterioration in ward patients: Systematic literature review', *Journal of Advanced Nursing*, vol. 65, no. 10, pp. 1992–2006.

Oermann, M.H., Conklin, J.L., Nicoll, L.H., Chinn, P.L., Ashton, K.S., Edie, A.H., Amarasekara, S. & Budinger, S.C., 2016, 'Study of predatory open access nursing journals', *Journal of Nursing Scholarship*, vol. 48, no. 6, pp. 624–632.

Paterno, M.T., McElroy, K. & Regan, M., 2016, 'Electronic fetal monitoring and caesarean birth: A scoping review', *Birth*, vol. 43, no. 4, pp. 277–284.

Peters, M.D.J., Godfrey, C.M., Khalil, H., McInerney, P., Parker, D. & Soares, C.B., 2015, 'Guidance for conducting systematic scoping reviews', *International Journal of Evidence-Based Healthcare*, vol. 13, pp. 141–146.

Peterson, J., Pearce, P.F., Ferguson, L.A. & Langford, C.A., 2016, 'Understanding scoping reviews: Definition, purpose and process', *Journal of the American Association of Nurse Practitioners*, vol. 29, pp. 12–16.

Porritt, K., Gomersall, J. & Lockwood, C., 2014, 'Study selection and critical appraisal', *American Journal of Nursing*, vol. 114, no. 6, pp. 47–52.

Robertson-Malt, S., 2014, 'Presenting and interpreting findings', *American Journal of Nursing*, vol. 114, no. 8, pp. 49–54.

Stern, C., Jordan, Z. & McArthur, A., 2014, 'Developing the review question and inclusion criteria', *American Journal of Nursing*, vol. 114, no. 4, pp. 53–56.

Thomas, A., Lubarsky, S., Durning, S.J. & Young, M.E., 2017, 'Knowledge synthesis in medical education: Demystifying scoping reviews', *Academic Medicine*, vol. 92, no. 2, pp. 161–166.

Timm, D.F., Banks, D.E. & McLarty, J., 2012, 'Critical appraisal process: Step-by-step', *Southern Medical Journal*, vol. 105, no. 3, pp. 144–148.

Umlauf, M.G., 2016, 'Predatory open access journals: Avoiding profiteers, wasted effort and fraud', *International Journal of Nursing Practice*, vol. 22, no. S1, pp. 3–4.

US National Library of Medicine, 2018, *Medical Subject Headings*, <www.nlm.nih.gov/mesh/>.

Williamson, K.M., 2009, 'Evidence-based practice: Critical appraisal of qualitative evidence', *Journal of the American Psychiatric Nurses Association*, vol. 15, no. 3, pp. 202–207.

CHAPTER 7

Ethics and research in nursing and midwifery

LEARNING OBJECTIVES

After working through this chapter, you should be able to:

- discuss the role of Human Research Ethics Committees
- describe the principles underpinning the ethical conduct of research
- identify researchers' responsibilities in ensuring their research is ethical
- identify bodies responsible for formulating policy in research ethics
- discuss issues relating to using web-based and social media sources for research.

KEY TERMS AND CONCEPTS

Approval processes, beneficence/non-maleficence, ethical principles, ethics, Human Research Ethics Committees, justice, research integrity, research merit, respect for persons

CASE STUDY OVERVIEW

Michael is the nurse unit manager in a busy medical ward. Current ward policy is that all patients have their vital signs recorded every four hours, regardless of their condition. He feels this is inefficient in terms of making best use of nursing staff's time, that it does not promote critical-thinking skills and that it is ineffective in detecting patient deterioration. He suggests that individualising frequency of vital signs measurement according to patient condition would be more effective. He proposes to undertake a randomised controlled trial comparing current practice with individualised practice to determine whether nurses' abilities to detect patient deterioration improves.

CHAPTER INTRODUCTION

It is vital that researchers protect the rights of the people they study. In health research in particular, the people who are the subjects, or the participants, of research are often in a state of vulnerability. Rules or guidelines to ensure that research is conducted ethically and that participants' rights are protected are a relatively recent development. In this chapter, we will examine the *governance of human research ethics*, including the approval and monitoring processes. We will discuss the *principles of ethical research* conduct and procedures by which researchers can ensure they are followed.

Development of ethical principles in research

The question of **ethics** in research gained widespread attention after the Second World War when the experiments conducted by Nazi doctors in concentration camps came to light. However, there have been many other instances where research participants have not been treated ethically, both before and since. The first guideline on the ethical conduct of research was produced in 1947, following the verdict in the so-called Doctors' Trial at Nuremberg, Germany, and is thus known as the **Nuremberg Code** (Shuster 1997). The code established ten principles for properly designed scientific studies involving humans and the treatment of research participants.

Building on this, in 1964, the World Medical Association (2013) produced its version of ethical research principles, in the **Declaration of Helsinki**, based on a framework of universal human rights. It was addressed primarily to physicians undertaking medical research, but anyone conducting research into people's health was encouraged to abide by it. The declaration is an evolving document, taking into account developments in medicine and health care and the need for more complex research. It has been amended several times. It is internationally accepted and forms the basis for all national guidelines.

In Australia, the ethical conduct of research is governed by the National

ethics
a discipline area concerned with moral values and conduct

Nuremberg Code
a set of ethical research principles developed in response to human experimentation during the Second World War

Declaration of Helsinki
a set of ethical research principles for human research developed by the World Medical Association

Health and Medical Research Council. Originally focused on medical research, the principles it has laid down now apply to any research involving humans, in any discipline. Principles and guidance are set out in the National Statement on Ethical Conduct in Human Research, or the National Statement (NHMRC 2007). Like the Declaration of Helsinki, it has been revised several times. All researchers conducting research with people are expected to have read this statement and to abide by its principles, as are bodies responsible for approving and monitoring research studies.

Human Research Ethics Committees

In Australia, the oversight of the ethical conduct of research involving people is the responsibility of bodies called **Human Research Ethics Committees** (HRECs). Similar systems exist in other countries but often have different names. The word *human* is included to distinguish the process from animal research, which has slightly different guiding principles and processes. HRECs are established in hospitals, universities and several other institutions. They are convened under standards set by the National Health and Medical Research Council and are registered with and report to the council. The composition of an HREC is mandated in the National Statement: there must be a minimum of eight people, with equal numbers of men and women, and at least a third of the members must be from outside the institution for which the research is being reviewed. Members must include healthcare professionals, pastoral care workers, a lawyer, lay people, and people with research expertise. Interestingly, it is desirable rather than mandatory for at least one member to have experience in ethical decision-making (NHMRC 2007).

Human Research Ethics Committee
a committee that oversees compliance of human research with ethical standards; also known as an HREC

ethical approval
a part of the research process that involves seeking formal approval from a Human Research Ethics Committee to conduct a study

The role of HRECs is to ensure that research undertaken within their institutions, or by people affiliated with them (usually employees, but also students in the case of universities), complies with ethical standards. They review research proposals and grant or deny approval for the research to be undertaken. They are also responsible for monitoring studies that have been approved, usually through annual reports submitted by researchers, though additional processes may be required in cases of high-risk research.

It should be noted that decisions about the ethics of conducting research are not always straightforward, and different HRECs do not always reach the same decisions. Ethical standards are not a set of rules to be followed mechanically. As the National Statement points out, application of the guidelines 'always requires, from each individual, deliberation on the values and principles, exercise of judgement, and an appreciation of context' (NHMRC 2007, p. 11).

ACTIVITY 7.1 Human Research Ethics Committees

1 Locate information about the HREC responsible for approving research in your institution.
2 Obtain the application form and read the questions, relating them to the principles of ethical conduct described below: *research merit and integrity, beneficence and non-maleficence, respect for persons* and *justice*.

Questions for consideration
• What are the procedures necessary for applying for ethical approval in your institution?
• What forms need to be completed?
• Are there different levels of approval for different types of research?
• Are all the ethical conduct principles listed above covered in the application form?
• Are there any questions on the form that do not relate to the principles?

Principles of ethical conduct of research

Ethical conduct of research continues to be underpinned by a framework of universal human rights. While the rights of participants in research are the primary concern, the rights of the wider community and of researchers themselves are also taken into account. The National Statement sets out four principles of ethical conduct: *research merit and integrity, beneficence and non-maleficence, respect for persons* and *justice* (NHMRC 2007).

Research merit and integrity

This principle is underpinned by the belief that research must be free from major flaws and carried out honestly. It should be obvious that research fraud and misconduct are unethical (even illegal in some cases); it may be less obvious that poor quality research can also have ethical implications. The rationale is that practice based on evidence that is unreliable, for whatever reason, is potentially dangerous (Moore et al. 2010).

The concept of **research merit** precludes research being undertaken for no good reason. It requires that there is potential benefit from any research; depending on the topic and the procedures involved, this could simply mean contributing to a body of knowledge. Researchers are required to provide full justification for their proposed research, including showing how it fits with what is already known (through a literature review). It is not ethical to continue researching a procedure or therapy if there is already strong evidence for or against its use. A component of research merit is ensuring that the research question can be answered and the potential benefit realised. This includes demonstrating that the design is appropriate to answer the question, that the sample size is appropriate (too small and the question may not be answered; too large and participants could be exposed to unnecessary risks), that the researchers have sufficient experience and qualifications to undertake the research and that necessary facilities and resources are available. All of these factors should be demonstrated in the research proposal.

research merit
an ethical principle requiring that a research study must have potential benefit and that this benefit can be realised

Research integrity means that research must be conducted and reported honestly. Violations of this tenet can include manipulating study procedures to make it more likely that a desired outcome is achieved, altering data, fabricating data, selective reporting of outcomes and fabricating entire studies (Moore et al. 2010). A number of codes of conduct have been developed to assist researchers in good research practice. The Australian Code for the Responsible Conduct of Research, jointly authored by the

research integrity
honesty in research conduct and reporting

National Health and Medical Research Council, the Australian Research Council and Universities Australia, sets out a number of principles and practices, including guidelines for data management and retention and standards for publication and dissemination of findings (NHMRC et al. 2018). An international standard called Good Clinical Practice has been developed specifically for 'activities concerning the conduct and reporting of clinical trials' (RCTs), but many of its principles can be applied more widely (ICH 2016). The Australian Therapeutic Goods Administration (TGA) has also produced documents intended for use in the conduct of clinical trials, particularly those involving medicines or medical devices (over which the TGA has some regulatory power); again, many of the guidelines have a wider application. The documents include the *Note for Guidance on Clinical Safety Data Management* and the *Australian Clinical Trial Handbook* (TGA, 2000, 2018). All guidelines emphasise the need for study procedures to be transparent and auditable and therefore carefully documented. Standards for recording and managing data to minimise the possibility of fraud are included. The guidelines mention standards for disseminating research findings, which have been further developed by the international Committee on Publication Ethics (or COPE). The standards include requirements for authors to declare any conflicts of interest and standards on what constitutes authorship (preventing 'honorary' authorship, and making all named authors responsible for the content of a paper).

Beneficence and non-maleficence

The principle of **beneficence** and **non-maleficence** is underpinned by the belief that people have the right not to be harmed. The requirement is that the likely benefits of research must outweigh any risk of harm or discomfort. The benefits may be to the participants themselves, to the wider community or to both. This principle is not just concerned with physical harm; participants can suffer emotional, psychological, financial, social or legal harm, depending on the purpose of the research. Researchers are responsible for assessing the known risks and designing research to minimise them. This could mean testing procedures beforehand to ensure their safety or taking

beneficence
to do good; in research, a study should aim to have good potential outcomes

non-maleficence
to do no harm; in research, a study should not cause harm to participants

steps to prevent harm. For example, financial harm may result if participants incur expenses as part of their role in the research; this can be avoided by reimbursing them for any expenditure. Any risks must be made known to potential participants. Researchers are also responsible for ensuring the welfare of participants during (and possibly after) the research. Procedures for managing potential risks and reporting any unintended outcomes must be built in to the research proposal.

In assessing risk, researchers and ethics committees have to take into account both the severity and the likelihood of the risk. *Severity* can be classified under the levels harm, discomfort and inconvenience:

- **Harm** Can range from extreme, such as major morbidity or even death, to relatively minor, such as temporary distress from reliving unpleasant experiences in an interview or experiencing unpleasant side-effects of medications.
- **Discomfort** Less serious than harm; it can be physical or emotional and may result from very minor side-effects of medications or stress from taking part in an interview or being observed at work, for example.
- **Inconvenience** Less serious again; it can occur with activities such as filling in a form or taking time to participate in research.

Likelihood is the possibility of adverse outcomes occurring. For example, there may be a very remote chance (say, 1 in 10,000) of major physical harm resulting from the study procedures. While this should not be discounted, it will most probably not be counted as a major risk. The possibility of discomfort could be very high (close to 100 per cent), and while this would probably be counted an acceptable risk, the researchers would still need a plan to manage it. Studies can be classed as *low risk* if the only likely adverse outcome is discomfort and as *negligible risk* if the only foreseeable risk is inconvenience. Ethics committees often have different procedures for each risk level.

In this chapter's case study, the outcome in Michael's proposed trial is patient deterioration, either detected by nurses and managed appropriately or not detected, with the consequent risk of a poor outcome for the patient. This constitutes harm. Even though this is a risk with current practice, it will be considered in assessing the risk of the study. Michael will have to argue that the study carries sufficient likely benefit to outweigh the potential for harm. Although he hopes that the new practice will reduce the number of patients whose deterioration is not detected, he does not know that it will do so (otherwise, there would be no point in doing the research), and there is a possibility that the opposite will happen: that the number will be increased. Because the severity of harm is high, Michael will need a plan for monitoring patient welfare during the study.

While risks to participants are the main concern of those overseeing research, in some situations the researchers themselves may be at risk as well. Physical harm can result from research procedures. Research carried out in the workplace is subject to usual health and safety regulations and should therefore require no additional precautions. However, if research is conducted outside the workplace—for instance, in field work or by going into participants' homes—a risk assessment for the researcher should be made and a plan put in place (Butler et al. 2017). Researchers can also be at risk of psychological or emotional harm if researching a sensitive topic; of social harm if, for example, their relationships are affected; and of academic or professional harm if their research findings are controversial.

ACTIVITY 7.2 Risks of research

The following case studies were discussed in Chapters 4 and 5.

1 Peter plans a quasi-experimental study to see if a nurse education program can improve person-centred care. He plans to measure person-centred care before and after the program to see if there is a difference. Two potential studies are suggested:
  • Person-centred care is measured by surveying patients to determine their satisfaction with care.
  • Person-centred care is measured by surveying nurses to determine the extent to which it is practised.

2 Stephanie proposes to measure person-centred care in her ward to determine how well it is practised. Two ways of doing this are suggested:
  • Nurses are observed in their practice, with the number of times they practise in a person-centred way noted.
  • Nurses are surveyed with the same tool as that used by Peter.
3 Jill plans to interview nurses on her ward to explore their understanding of person-centred care.

Questions for consideration

• What risks do you consider there are to participants in each of these scenarios?
• How might the researchers manage the risks?
• Are there any risks to the researchers?

Respect for persons

This principle is underpinned by the belief that people have a right to **self-determination.** The principle is sometimes referred to as **autonomy** but is actually broader than this. The basic concept is of **informed consent**: that research should not be carried out on people without their knowledge and permission. This is a legal as well as an ethical imperative. Note that there is no such thing as uninformed consent—no one can be deemed to consent to something of which they have no knowledge or understanding.

Ensuring that participants are informed requires researchers to provide full disclosure on what is involved in taking part in the research, including any risks that may be involved, as well as the consequences of not taking part. This latter point is very important when testing or evaluating new practices, such as new therapies; patients need to know what care they will receive if they decline to be in the study. A minimum requirement is that information be provided in writing, in a document called a *participant information statement.* Information must be provided in a language and at a level that people can readily understand. Researchers must make every effort to overcome any other factors that

self-determination
the freedom to make one's own decisions

autonomy
the right to exercise one's will

informed consent
a person's agreement to be included in research based on full disclosure of what is involved

may limit people's ability to understand the material. For example, people in a highly stressful situation—such as sudden illness—are less likely to be able to assimilate information. Researchers can help by providing time for people to consider whether they want to take part and opportunities for them to ask questions about the research.

When they have sufficient information to make an informed decision, potential participants are asked to provide their consent to take part in the research. Consent can be provided in a number of ways. In most research in which the researchers and participants have direct contact, written—signed—consent is required. This is the equivalent of signing a legal document. Occasionally, verbal consent may be sufficient; this is likely to occur in low-risk situations. Sometimes, consent can be implied by the participant's continuing with the study procedures. The commonest scenario of **implied consent** is that of a survey, where filling out and returning or submitting a questionnaire can be interpreted as the person's consenting to take part in the study.

implied consent
agreement to take part can be assumed by an activity, such as filling out a questionnaire

In some studies, it can be difficult or even impossible to obtain informed consent at the time that potential participants need to be enrolled. Examples include emergency situations involving unconscious patients, and women in the second stage of labour. Sometimes, seeking formal consent can impose an unnecessary risk or burden on participants. Several alternative methods for obtaining consent have been developed to enable research to be undertaken in these situations. One is **deferred** or **retrospective consent**. This method was used in a large medical study to evaluate whether saline or albumin should be used for fluid resuscitation in critically ill patients (SAFE Study Investigators 2004). At the time the fluid had to be given, the patients were by definition too ill to provide consent. Eligible patients were therefore enrolled without consent, then, later, either they or their next of kin were told about the study and asked if they wanted to remain in it. If they did not, they were removed from the study and their data deleted. Another alternative is the **opt out** method. This method was described by Lam and

deferred or retrospective consent
formal consent for data to be used after those data have been collected

opt out consent
a mechanism whereby people refuse consent to take part in research, or for information about them to be used in research, before they become eligible for inclusion; if they do not take up this option they will be included automatically

East (2015) in regard to a study to determine whether measuring lactate in fetuses who become distressed during labour could lead to a reduction in the incidence of caesarean section. It was deemed that at the time when the decision to participate would need to be made, the mothers would not be in a good position to understand the information and provide informed consent. Therefore, they were told about the study when they were in early labour and given the opportunity to opt out at that stage. If they did not opt out, they were enrolled into the study if and when they became eligible. In other circumstances, the need to obtain consent can be waived altogether, although this is quite controversial. The National Statement provides guidelines for the application of all these strategies (NHMRC 2007).

Specific guidelines have been developed for the protection of populations deemed to be vulnerable, including those who are unable to provide consent for themselves. This category includes people who are unconscious, people who are mentally impaired, and children, all of whom are protected by legislation determining who can consent on their behalf. Pregnant women and fetuses are also numbered among the vulnerable populations, as are some ethnic minorities. In Australia, we have specific guidelines for research involving Aboriginal and Torres Strait Islander peoples (NHMRC 2003).

ACTIVITY 7.3 Informed consent

In our case study, patients in Michael's ward are an ethnically diverse group, and many have limited English-language skills. Moreover, a large proportion of patients have low literacy and numeracy skills.

Questions for consideration
- What challenges do these factors present in gaining informed consent?
- What strategies could Michael use to ensure consent is truly informed?

Another important point about consent is that it must be freely given; that is, people must not be **coerced** into taking part. The information

coercion
the unethical process of pressurising someone to participate in research

given to potential participants must always include a statement to the effect that participation is voluntary and that declining to participate will not result in any adverse effects—for example, patients' medical care will not be affected in any way. However, this statement may be insufficient: people may still feel pressured to take part. This is particularly the case if there is an unequal relationship between researchers and potential participants or if researchers are in a position of authority over potential participants. Examples of unequal relationships include health professionals and patients in their direct care, employers and employees, managers and subordinates, and teachers and students.

ACTIVITY 7.4 Clinical relationships

In the case study in Chapter 5, Jill, the unit manager on a busy medical-surgical unit, plans to undertake a qualitative study with the nurses in her ward, because she is concerned that the nursing care is not person-centred; that is, she perceives there is a deficit in the care being given.

Questions for consideration
- What ethical concerns might be raised by the relationship between Jill and her staff?
- What strategies could Jill employ to overcome these concerns?
- Is there a possibility of an unequal relationship in the research?

Also underpinning this principle is people's right to privacy. Every state and territory in Australia has its own privacy legislation, and researchers need to be aware of, and comply with, the relevant laws. They include ensuring that data are securely stored both during and after a study, so that unauthorised persons do not have access to them; not revealing information that participants want kept **confidential**; and usually not revealing in reports any information that could identify the participants. The last of these requirements can extend to institutions—for example, not revealing the name of a hospital where the research was carried out. The most complete protection of identity is conferred by **anonymity**, in which the researchers do not know who the participants are. This is possible in many surveys but rarely in other types of research. It should be noted that if researchers promise participants that they will be anonymous, written consent—which requires people's names to be recorded—cannot be requested. This is the reason that implied consent is acceptable in this situation.

confidentiality
the protection of information that a research participant does not wish to be made public; this can include, but is not limited to, concealment of their identity

anonymity
the state of a research participant's identity being unknown to researchers

Justice

The principle of **justice** is underpinned by the belief that people have a right to be treated fairly. It requires that the following conditions are met:

justice
the fair treatment of research participants

- Recruitment procedures are fair. This includes taking steps to ensure that anyone who might benefit from taking part in the study has the opportunity to do so. One reason for the requirement for registration of clinical trials is to enable people to search the registry to find out if there are any studies relevant to them.
- Participants are not exploited.
- Study procedures are fair to all participants and do not place an undue burden on any specific group. For example, if some people are required to travel long distances to take part in a study, they might either decide not to take part (thus missing out on any potential benefit), or they might take part but then be disadvantaged financially.
- Any benefits of participating in research are fairly distributed.
- Access to benefits of research findings is fair.
- Research outcomes are made available to all participants.

ACTIVITY 7.5 Exploring research ethics

Find a research report on any topic of interest to you.

Questions for consideration
- What information is included in the report about ethical issues? For example, is approval mentioned? Do the authors indicate how they addressed ethical concerns? Do they mention consent?
- Can you identify any ethical issues that are not mentioned?
- Do you consider that the authors have addressed ethical issues and their management in sufficient detail? If not, what other details would you like to have seen?

RESEARCH EXAMPLE 7.1 Ethical issues in collecting data by observation

Early-warning scoring systems to detect patient deterioration are routinely used in many healthcare facilities and depend on timely and accurate vital signs monitoring. As discussed in Chapter 6, Cardona-Morell et al. (2016) conducted a study by observation to explore monitoring practices of 42 nurses. The researchers followed the participating nurses throughout the course of their work, during times of day when vital signs were usually measured, and recorded the details of any interactions the nurses had with patients. They observed 441 nurse–patient interactions, of which just over half involved taking of vital signs. The researchers found that the minimum five vital signs measures required by health policy were taken in only 6–21 per cent of these instances of vital signs monitoring. They concluded that this prevalence of incomplete sets of vital signs could limit identification of deterioration in patients.

M. Cardona-Morrell, M. Prgomet, R. Lake, M. Nicholson, R. Harrison, J. Long, J. Westbrook, J. Braithwaite & K. Hillman, 2016, 'Vital signs monitoring and nurse–patient interaction: A qualitative observational study of hospital practice', *International Journal of Nursing Studies*, vol. 56, pp. 9–16.

Questions for consideration

- What ethical issues could be of concern in this study design?
- How would these issues be addressed to ensure the ethical conduct of research and patient safety, bearing in mind that the patients were not the study participants?

RESEARCH EXAMPLE 7.2 Ethical issues in collecting data by survey

Patient assessment, including vital signs monitoring, is an essential role of nurses and midwives, to detect and act upon deterioration in a patient's condition. Osborne et al. (2015) conducted a survey among all nurses and midwives in acute care areas of one hospital to examine how often nurses and midwives used physical assessment skills and to identify factors that influenced their actual assessments. Two established survey instruments were used, containing 179 questions in total. Eligible participants were identified by the nurse unit manager on each ward and were sent a survey package in the internal mail. An electronic version of the survey was made available on the hospital intranet for those who preferred to respond using this method.

S. Osborne, C. Douglas, C. Reid, L. Jones & G. Gardner, 2015, 'The primacy of vital signs—acute care nurses' and midwives' use of physical assessment skills: A cross sectional study', *International Journal of Nursing Studies*, vol. 52, pp. 951–962.

Questions for consideration

- What are the ethical issues in this study?
- What procedures should the researchers follow to ensure compliance with all the principles of ethical research conduct?

Internet and social media use in nursing and midwifery research

Many health professionals, including nurses and midwives, seek to use the internet and social media to access data for research. While it may be tempting to engage in collecting data from such sources, due to the ready availability of extensive pools of data, Lunnay et al. (2015) suggest that researchers need to be clear about the benefits of approaching social media for research activity. From an ethical perspective, having readily available research data raises a number of issues, and HRECs are increasingly having to consider applications proposing to use such sources. One issue is that data are potentially identifiable; for example, if taken from Facebook posts, data could be linked back to a person whose identity may be revealed. Also, people usually post to social media sites for personal reasons but not for the purpose of their posts being used for research purposes. Hence, they probably have not provided consent for the use of their posts, even though they are in the public domain.

ACTIVITY 7.6 Using social media sources in research

Think about your own social media use.

Questions for consideration
- Is there content that you post that could be used as research data?
- How might you feel if you were to see your posts directly used in research studies?
- What could be the potential benefits of using internet and social media content as data sources, particularly in nursing and midwifery research?

CHAPTER SUMMARY

Protection of both research participants and researchers is fundamental to good research practice. Ethical standards for conducting research have been established internationally and are governed locally. These standards are based on four guiding principles: research merit and integrity, beneficence and non-maleficence, respect for persons and justice. In this chapter, processes for the approval and monitoring of ethical conduct of research have been discussed. Finally, the area of ethical issues surrounding research using the internet or social media sources have been explored.

CHAPTER REVIEW QUESTIONS

- What institution is responsible for providing guidance and advice on ethical conduct of research in Australia?
- What is the role of Human Research Ethics Committees?
- What is meant by each of the following:
  —research merit and integrity
  —beneficence and non-maleficence
  —respect for persons
  —justice?
- What procedures can researchers follow to ensure ethical principles are upheld?
- What ethical issues may arise in research using the internet or social media as data sources?

QUESTIONS FOR DISCUSSION

- Why is ethics so important for research in health care?
- How can you determine whether research evidence has been generated ethically?
- What are the implications for nursing and midwifery if research is not ethical?
- How could we effectively use the internet or social media for meaningful nursing and midwifery research?

QUESTIONS FOR PERSONAL REFLECTION

- What have you learnt from this chapter about best practice in conducting research ethically?
- How will this impact on your reading of research reports?

USEFUL WEB RESOURCES

Committee on Publication Ethics <https://publicationethics.org>
National Health and Medical Research Council on ethical issues <www.nhmrc.gov.au/ health-ethics/ethical-issues-and-further-resources>
National Health and Medical Research Council on good clinical practice in Australia <www.australianclinicaltrials.gov.au/researchers/ good-clinical-practice-gcp-australia>

REFERENCES AND FURTHER READING

Bowrey, S. & Thompson, J., 2014, 'Nursing research: Ethics, consent and good practice', *Nursing Times*, vol. 110, no. 1/3, pp. 20–23.

Butler, A., Copnell, B. & Hall, H., 2017, 'Researching people who are bereaved: Managing risks to participants and researchers', *Nursing Ethics*, doi: 10.1177/0969733017695656.

Cardona-Morrell, M., Prgomet, M., Lake, R., Nicholson, M., Harrison, R., Long, J., Westbrook, J., Braithwaite, J. & Hillman, K., 2016, 'Vital signs monitoring and nurse–patient interaction: A qualitative observational study of hospital practice', *International Journal of Nursing Studies*, vol. 56, pp. 9–16.

Doody, O. & Noonan, M., 2016, 'Nursing research ethics, guidance and application in practice', *British Journal of Nursing*, vol. 25, no. 14, pp. 803–807.

ICH, 2016, *Integrated Addendum to ICH E6 (R1): Guideline for good clinical practice E6(R2)*, <www.tga.gov.au/publication/note-guidance-good-clinical-practice>.

Ingham-Broomfield, R., 2017, 'A nurses' guide to ethical considerations and the process for ethical approval of nursing research', *Australian Journal of Advanced Nursing*, vol. 35, no. 1, pp. 40–47.

International Council for Harmonisation of Technical Requirements for Pharmaceuticals for Human Use *see* ICH

Lam, L. & East, C., 2015, 'Evaluation of a novel opt-out consent process involving pregnant women', *Australian Nursing and Midwifery Journal*, vol. 22, no. 9, p. 43.

Lunnay, B., Borlagdan, J., McNaughton, D. & Ward, P., 2015, 'Ethical use of social media to facilitate qualitative research', *Qualitative Health Research*, vol. 25, no. 1, pp. 99–109.

Mahon, P.Y., 2014, 'Internet research and ethics: Transformative issues in nursing education research', *Journal of Professional Nursing*, vol. 30, pp. 124–129.

Milton, C.L., 2013, 'The ethics of research', *Nursing Science Quarterly*, vol. 26, no. 1, pp. 20–23.

Moore, R.A., Derry, S. & McQuay, H.J., 2010, 'Fraud or flawed: Adverse impact of fabricated or poor quality research', *Anaesthesia*, vol. 65, no. 4, pp. 327–330, doi: 10.1111/j.1365-2044.2010.06295.x.

National Health and Medical Research Council *see* NHMRC

NHMRC, 2003, *Values and Ethics: Guidelines for ethical conduct in Aboriginal and Torres Strait Islander health research*, Canberra: Commonwealth of Australia.

NHMRC, 2007, *National Statement on Ethical Conduct in Human Research*, updated May 2015, Canberra: Commonwealth of Australia.

NHMRC, Australian Research Council & Universities Australia, 2018, *Australian Code for the Responsible Conduct of Research*, Canberra: Commonwealth of Australia.

Osborne, S., Douglas, C., Reid, C., Jones, L. & Gardner, G., 2015, 'The primacy of vital signs—acute care nurses' and midwives' use of physical assessment skills: A cross sectional study', *International Journal of Nursing Studies*, vol. 52, pp. 951–962.

SAFE Study Investigators, 2004, 'A comparison of albumin and saline for fluid resuscitation in the intensive care unit', *New England Journal of Medicine*, vol. 350, no. 22, pp. 2247–2256, doi: 10.1056/NEJMoa040232.

Shuster, E., 1997, 'Fifty years later: The significance of the Nuremberg Code', *New England Journal of Medicine*, vol. 337, pp. 1436–1440.

Therapeutic Goods Administration, 2000, *Note for Guidance on Clinical Safety Data Management: Definitions and standards for expedited reporting*, Canberra: Commonwealth of Australia.

Therapeutic Goods Administration, 2018, *Australian Clinical Trial Handbook v2.0*, Canberra: Commonwealth of Australia.

World Medical Association, 2013, *Declaration of Helsinki: Ethical principles for medical research involving human subjects*, <www.wma.net/policies-post/wma-declaration-of-helsinki-ethical-principles-for-medical-research-involving-human-subjects/>.

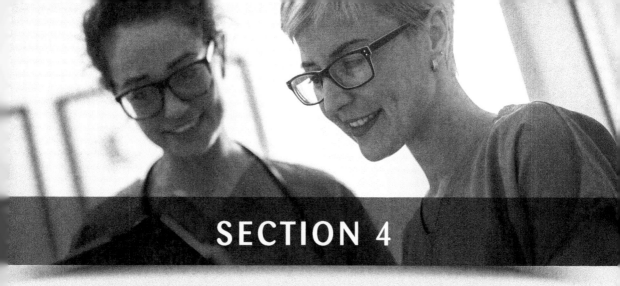

SECTION 4

HOW DO I USE EVIDENCE TO INFORM MY PRACTICE?

The previous sections in this book have explored the nature of evidence in nursing and midwifery, where and how to source it and making sense of it. In this section, we take the next step, exploring how evidence can be applied to nursing and midwifery to make a difference to our care of people. Knowledge translation—the translation of research-based evidence into practice—is imperative if that evidence is to make a real difference.

Chapter 8 specifically explores the processes by which knowledge can be translated into practice. It explores how nurses and midwives can question their practice to enhance the care they deliver.

An important skill for nurses and midwives is the writing of literature reviews. In Chapter 6, we introduced the systematic and scoping reviews as examples. Chapter 9 examines the writing of literature reviews, which you may be required to produce as a student or for colleagues in clinical practice, and how to approach it.

CHAPTER 8

Applying evidence in practice

LEARNING OBJECTIVES

After working through this chapter, you should be able to:

- discuss the importance of evidence-based practice in nursing and midwifery
- identify who is responsible for the translation of knowledge to practice
- outline the role of clinical practice guidelines and clinical audit in evidence-based practice
- discuss some of the models that can be used to guide evidence implementation
- discuss ways to evaluate the implementation of new evidence into practice
- identify factors impacting on the implementation of evidence into practice.

KEY TERMS AND CONCEPTS

Action research, evidence implementation, implementation science, knowledge translation, realist evaluation

CASE STUDY OVERVIEW

John is a clinical nurse specialist on a busy medical-surgical ward. He is concerned about a recent rise in medication errors in the ward. He decides to examine the available evidence in the area and explore the current practices in the ward to see if they are impacting on the rising error rates.

CHAPTER INTRODUCTION

Evidence-based practice is an important part of nursing and midwifery. Research is growing rapidly; however, much of the evidence generated may never be translated into practice. Just as research needs to be conducted systematically and thoroughly, so too does the translation of new knowledge into clinical practice. This requires a process for implementing the evidence, as well as for evaluating its effectiveness at the local level. In this chapter, we will explore the process for doing that, through the concept of **knowledge translation**, models and processes for implementing evidence into practice and strategies for evaluating its impact.

Responsibility for knowledge translation

knowledge translation
the process of translating research knowledge into practice contexts

One of the challenges facing researchers and clinicians is the divide between the generation and the implementation into practice of research knowledge. Whose responsibility is the implementation of new knowledge into clinical practice? The only people who can realistically be responsible for this are clinicians, regardless of their area of practice. They are providing the care and as such, have the contact with the people receiving the care informed by the research. That being said, researchers have a responsibility to be doing the types of research that clinicians need to inform their practice. As we highlighted in Chapter 1, the Nurses and Midwifery Board of Australia standards and competencies require nurses and midwives to use evidence to support their care, reinforcing their roles and responsibilities in this regard. In addition, the Australian Nursing and Midwifery Federation has developed its own policy for research and evidence-based practice.

It is widely recognised that it is not appropriate for decisions about care delivery to be based upon what has been traditionally done or to be made according to the preference of the care provider (Spruce 2015). Rather, care decisions need to be driven by the best available research evidence. While this sounds logical, many challenges have been faced by nurses and midwives in applying evidence-based practice and hence in the delivery of best-practice care.

ACTIVITY 8.1 Responsibility for knowledge translation

In this chapter's case study, John is concerned about the rising medication error rate on his ward.

Questions for consideration
- Who in the ward is responsible for the review of new evidence regarding medication administration practices?
- What factors have influenced your views on this allocation of responsibility for evidence application?

ACTIVITY 8.2 Reflecting on knowledge translation

Think of a clinical practice area where you have recent experience.

Questions for consideration
- Was knowledge translation considered to be important?
- Whose role was specifically related to knowledge translation?
- Who else had some responsibility for knowledge translation in that area?
- From where was new knowledge sourced to inform practice change?
- Did you observe a clinical audit or use of clinical practice guidelines informing practice?

Questioning clinical practice

In order to recognise a need for new evidence to support practice, it is necessary to question the existing practice. It is not sufficient to continue traditional practice just because it has always been done that way. It may not be delivering the best practice to those people who are receiving care.

It is essential to constantly question clinical practice. Some questions that can be asked are:

- What is the current practice?
- Why is it undertaken that way?
- What evidence is it based upon?
- Is newer evidence available?
- Is a change in practice feasible in this clinical setting?

However, questioning clinical practice can be challenging, particularly in areas where the same staff have been working and delivering care together in the same ways for many years. Implementing practice change cannot be effectively undertaken by one person; rather, a team-based approach is crucial to implementing and maintaining any new practice. Garnering support for change will be important for ensuring its relevance to practice and the potential for successful implementation.

Sources of evidence for practice

We have closely examined the role of research literature in informing evidence-based practice. However, there are other sources from which credible knowledge to inform clinical practice can be drawn, as described below.

Clinical practice guidelines

These are guidelines for clinical practice that have been developed based on the best available evidence, so a lot of the work around sourcing and evaluating evidence has already been conducted. **Clinical practice guidelines** allow healthcare professionals to make sound decisions and deliver optimal care in specific circumstances. Organisations, such as hospitals, often develop clinical practice guidelines specifically in their own settings. In addition, the National Health and Medical Research Council has established the Australian Clinical Practice Guidelines Portal, where over 2000 guidelines developed by organisations can be accessed and are

clinical practice guidelines
guidelines for informing clinical practice developed from best available evidence

available to others (NHMRC 2017). Any newly submitted guidelines are evaluated using the following questions:

- Is the guideline evidence based?
- Is the guideline Australian?
- Is the guideline current?
- Is the guideline freely available?
- Is a funding statement included in the guideline?
- Was the guideline developed in a transparent manner with potential conflicts of interest stated?
- Was the guideline developed under the auspices of a professional college or association? (NHMRC 2017)

In the United Kingdom, the National Institute for Health and Care Excellence (or NICE) has an extensive bank of clinical practice guidelines and audits <www.nice.org.uk> and contains a large number of clinical practice guidelines specific to nursing.

Clinical audit

Clinical audits are commonly used in health care to measure aspects of performance. They form an important aspect of clinical governance and quality improvement. They can be conducted at ward or organisation level. Benjamin (2008) presents clinical audit as a cyclical process with five stages, as reproduced in the list below, to which we have added brief explanations:

clinical audit
a review of current practice and performance against best available evidence

1 **Preparing for audit** Identifying the problem and local resources needed for the audit.
2 **Selecting criteria for audit review** Deciding what is being measured and the performance standard desired.
3 **Measuring level of performance** Collecting data and comparing it with the desired level of performance.
4 **Making improvements** Implementing necessary change.
5 **Sustaining improvements** Monitoring (including potential repeat audits) and sustaining change (Benjamin 2008).

ACTIVITY 8.3 Questioning clinical practice

Think about a clinical skill that you are familiar with and how you have seen that skill performed in practice. Use the questions at the beginning of this section to conduct an evaluation of the skill as you saw it in practice.

Questions for consideration

- Was that practice based on best available evidence?
- How might a clinical audit be employed to improve it?

Implementing evidence into practice

The implementation of new evidence into clinical practice requires a team-based, structured approach. Spruce (2015) suggests a number of practical steps that provide a logical way to approach practice change. Once again, we have added explanations to Spruce's steps in the list below:

- **Form a project team and identify the scope of the project** The successful implementation of evidence into clinical practice requires a team approach. The team needs to agree to the scope of the implementation and its evaluation. It is also important to consider the inclusion of other health professionals in the team who may be impacted by the change.
- **Identify the evidence** A search for relevant evidence is a key component of the process. With librarians' expertise in search strategies, it is worth considering the inclusion of a librarian in the team, particularly for this aspect.
- **Conduct a rapid review** A rapid review requires skimming the accessed resources and summarising the evidence to identify the key research papers that meet the project needs.
- **Assign articles** Spruce recommends assigning articles throughout the team for the purpose of conducting a quality appraisal.

- **Use appraisal tools** Having consistency across the appraisal process is fundamental to ensuring the best evidence is utilised. This requires using a quality assessment appraisal tool (see Chapter 6).
- **Make practice recommendations** From the quality appraisal, the team can work out the best practices for the local setting.
- **Identify implementation strategies** Implementation strategies need to be carefully thought through, as they will directly affect the success of the implementation. These should include a number of considerations:
  - steps involved in the project
  - whether approval from management or a Human Research Ethics Committee is required. The latter is important if there is a plan to publish the findings
  - staff preparation and education regarding implementation of the intervention
  - necessary resources—for example, equipment or evaluation tools
  - whether a pilot test or study is required before completely introducing the intervention
  - managing feedback
  - identifying who will take the lead and champion the work. (Spruce 2015, pp. 108–109)

ACTIVITY 8.4 Evidence implementation

In our case study, John is concerned about the rising medication error rate on his ward. He uses a questioning approach to consider the current medication administration practice in the ward, discovering that many practices are not evidence based. He decides to review clinical practice guidelines and to undertake a clinical audit. From these, he confirms that current medication management practices are not evidence based or ensuring the delivery of optimal quality care. He sets about forming a team to work on implementing new evidence-based practice.

Questions for consideration

- What skills might be needed in the team?
- Who might be key people in the team?
- What else needs consideration?
- What should John do once he has the team together?

RESEARCH EXAMPLE 8.1 Examining evidence-based nursing and midwifery practice

Fairbrother et al. (2016) conducted a survey to assess the needs and skills for, and barriers to, evidence-based practice in one local health district in regional New South Wales, Australia. A total of 169 senior nurses and midwives completed the survey. Findings indicated that these nurses and midwives relied on subjective information from patients and their own knowledge, rather than published evidence, to support their practice. Availability of, as well as ability to read, research reports was considered a barrier. In addition, time was a reported barrier to implementing evidence-based practice. The researchers concluded that there was a need for capacity-building interventions to develop staff skills with regard to evidence-based practice.

G. Fairbrother, A. Cashin, R. Conway & I. Graham, 2016, 'Evidence based nursing and midwifery practice in a regional Australian healthcare setting: Behaviours, skills and barriers', *Collegian*, vol. 23, pp. 29–37.

Questions for consideration

- Do you think the findings of this study might be similar elsewhere, that is, transferable?
- How might these findings be used to develop evidence-based practice?

Evidence-based practice models

Numerous models have been developed and employed by nurses and midwives to facilitate the successful application of evidence to their practice. In this section, we will take a look at a selection of these models.

Johns Hopkins Nursing Evidence-Based Practice Model

The Johns Hopkins Nursing Evidence-Based Practice Model (or JHNEBP) provides a structured decision-making approach to applying evidence to clinical nursing practice. It uses a three-step process referred to as *PET*: *practice question*, *evidence* and *translation*. Within the model are nineteen steps to guide evidence-based practice. Various tools are provided to guide teams through the process, from development of the initial question to dissemination of findings arising from the process (Johns Hopkins Medicine 2017).

Promoting Action on Research Implementation in Health Services

In 1998, Kitson et al. developed the Promoting Action on Research Implementation in Health Services (or PARIHS) framework. This approach to knowledge translation is underpinned by the concept that 'successful implementation of research in practice is a function of the relation between the nature of the evidence, the context in which the proposed change is to be implemented and the mechanisms by which the change is facilitated'. The authors introduced the formula:

$$SI = f(E, C, F),$$

where successful implementation (SI) is a function (f) of evidence (E), context (C) and facilitation (F). In the model, there is an emphasis on the facilitator, who works with people to see the need for change and in making the change happen (Kitson et al. 1998, p. 150).

Advancing Research and Clinical Practice through Close Collaboration

The Advancing Research and Clinical Practice through Close Collaboration (or ARCC) model takes a very different, behavioural approach to effective implementation of evidence into practice, being underpinned by control theory and cognitive behavioural theory. This model makes four key assumptions:

1   Barriers and facilitators to evidence-based practice exist for individuals in the healthcare systems in which they work.

2   Barriers to evidence-based practice need to be managed and mitigated, while facilitators need to be put into place.

3   There is a need to strengthen clinicians' beliefs regarding the value of evidence-based practice and their confidence to use it.

4   There needs to be a culture of evidence-based practice in the work-place. (Melnyk & Fineout-Overholt 2010, pp. 170–171)

Within the model, there are six key tenets that need to be in place for evidence implementation to be successful:

1   Inquiry is a daily part of the healthcare environment.
2   The overall goal is achieving quality outcomes.
3   Processes are in place to support the achievement of optimal outcomes.
4   There is transparency in outcome and process data.
5   Clinicians are able to function as autonomous change agents.
6   Health care is delivered in a dynamic environment. (Melnyk & Fineout-Overholt 2010, pp. 176–177)

ACTIVITY 8.5 Exploring an evidence-based practice model

1 Select an evidence-based practice model, either from those above or another you are aware of.
2 Search for some literature where that model has been utilised.
3 Summarise how the model was used in evidence implementation.

Questions for consideration

• How successful was the implementation?
• Were there any challenges reported by the authors in applying the model?

Evaluation of practice change

The implementation of new evidence is not complete just with the practice change. It is important to know if the change makes a difference and whether it is appropriate. One of the limitations regularly stated in research papers is that the findings may not be generalisable to any other population beyond that included in the study. Whenever new evidence is being implemented, there may be differences in the practice setting that influence its usefulness. Hence, evaluation of the implementation of new knowledge is vital to ensure it makes a positive change. Such evaluation can form a type of research study in its own right—hence, again, the need for nurses and midwives to possess some research knowledge and skills. Evaluation might constitute a range of data collection tools, such as questionnaires, interviews and observations. There are numerous approaches to evaluating evidence implementation. In this section, we will look at two approaches, *action research* and *realist evaluation*, which both develop and implement new evidence for practice.

Action research

Action research is a practical qualitative research approach that has been used for many years in nursing and midwifery, among other disciplines. The *action* nature of this approach makes it unique in practice change. It is known as a *participatory* approach to research, because the participants are actively involved as members of the research team, helping to guide its progress as well as to allow participants to be empowered. According to Casey et al. (2017), action research 'aims to create and/or add to existing theoretical and practice knowledge'.

> **action research**
> a cyclical research approach designed to facilitate change through empowering participants

In recent years, we have seen the evolution of **implementation science**. Eccles and Mittman (2006) define this as 'the scientific study of methods to promote the systematic uptake of research findings and other evidence-based practices (EBP) into routine practice'. These authors point out that

> **implementation science**
> an emerging scientific field examining implementation of existing evidence into practice and policy

implementation science is different from action research in that its focus rests on the implementation of existing evidence to inform healthcare practice and policy, while action research develops, as well as implements, evidence.

Action research occurs in a cyclical process. There are four steps involved in this approach that may be repeated many times as the research unfolds. In each step, there may be different elements of data generated, depending on what is being explored:

1   **Planning** The team involved in the change works together to develop a plan for the next step. The key is involving and empowering each member to take their part in making decisions and contributing to the research direction. In the case of a new practice being implemented, the group determines what the change is, and when and how it is to be implemented, managed and evaluated.
2   **Action** The plan from the previous step is implemented. In the case of a practice change, it is in this stage that the new practice is trialled as the group has previously determined.
3   **Observation** The group works together to monitor the implementation of the plan. This includes deciding whether there are changes required or other issues arising that need to be considered.
4   **Reflection** The group reflects on the plan, reviewing its implementation and any other considerations. The plans for the next cycle of the action research process are initiated.

The number of cycles in action research studies will vary. However, generally, they have a timeframe determined by the research group.

RESEARCH EXAMPLE 8.2 Action research in implementation
of evidence-based practice

In one ward of a rural hospital in the Netherlands, Friesen-Storms et al. (2014) conducted action research to empower nurses to use evidence-based practice to develop a patient discharge protocol. Over a 24-month period, they conducted a program of developing and implementing evidence-based practice through cycles of planning, acting, observing and reflecting. Participants included not only the nurses but other key stakeholders—for example, patients and their caregivers. Results of the study indicated that best practice in patient discharge was being implemented in the ward. There were reported barriers—for example, nurses' knowledge of evidence-based practice, some lingering negativity, time factors and English proficiency (as much of the research literature was written in that language). However, the researchers also reported facilitators: the nurses held a desire to provide high-quality care to patients, they were open to innovation, and they reported that the research stimulated their critical thinking around evidence-based practice and patient care.

J.H.H.M. Friesen-Storms, A. Moser, S. van der Loo, A.J.H.M. Beurskens & G.J.J.W. Bours, 2014, 'Systematic implementation of evidence-based practice in a clinical nursing setting: A participatory action research project', *Journal of Clinical Nursing*, vol. 24, pp. 57–68.

Questions for consideration
- Why was action research an appropriate choice for this study?
- Why was it a more appropriate approach than another such as phenomenology or grounded theory?
- How can findings from action research such as this lead to enhanced care delivery?
- What might be the benefits of using action research in nursing and midwifery practice settings?

ACTIVITY 8.6 Action research

Think of a clinical practice that could be changed using an action research approach.

Questions for consideration
- What aspects of the practice need to change?
- What is the context in which the research will occur?
- Who will need to be involved?
- How many cycles might be needed? What will these entail?

Data collection in action research

During the process of action research, a range of data can be collected. Their purpose is to provide evidence to support the practice change. Data can be quantitative (such as questionnaires, experimental studies, auditing of clinical documentation) or qualitative (interviews, observations, focus groups) in nature, or both, and often various approaches are employed. All will aid in evaluating the effectiveness or impact of the practice change.

Challenges in action research

It would be easy to conduct an implementation process and call it an action research study. However, as with any research study, action research needs to be conducted in a rigorous and defendable way. Munten et al. (2010) reviewed 21 action research studies that had been performed in nursing and found that many did not report on their implementation strategies. They concluded that action research showed promise in the implementation of evidence into nursing practice but there was a need for action researchers to provide clear and detailed descriptions of their implementation strategies. This is important in order to publish findings from action research studies and for others to utilise the evidence generated in their own clinical settings.

Realist evaluation

Realist evaluation is an increasingly popular approach, particularly in health care, to examine the nature of programs and how they work, for the purpose of refining or testing theory. It translates research approaches into the domains of policy and practice that stresses the importance of stakeholders in the process. The methodology varies but can employ qualitative or quantitative methods, depending on the evaluation (Pawson & Tilley 1997, 2004).

realist evaluation
an approach to evaluating programs and how they work

The process of realist evaluation involves four main concepts, as outlined by Pawson and Tilley (2004); we have once again added explanations to their list:

1 **Mechanism** The nature of programs or interventions that actually bring about effects.
2 **Context** The context in which programs are introduced or delivered.
3 **Outcome patterns** The outcomes of the program, both intended and unintended.
4 **Context mechanism outcome pattern configuration** The way in which all concepts work together overall; also called CMOC.

Realist evaluation, like action research, is conducted in a four-stage research cycle. Our explanations follow the stages as listed by Pawson and Tilley:

1 **Hypothesis** Information is accessed and theory formulated about what in the program 'works for whom in what circumstances'.
2 **Data collection** Data are collected on the mechanisms, contexts and outcomes of the program and can be diverse, with information drawn from such sources as questionnaires, interviews and observations.
3 **Data analysis** Data are analysed to explore outcome patterns and examine which of these can be explained through the initial theory and which cannot.
4 **Theory testing** Understandings of the context mechanism outcome pattern configuration are revised and it is decided if another cycle is needed. (Pawson & Tilley 2004, p. 24)

ACTIVITY 8.7 Realist evaluation

Think about the clinical practice that you used in Activity 8.6.

Questions for consideration
• Could realist evaluation be used to implement and evaluate the required change?
• If not, why not?

RESEARCH EXAMPLE 8.3 Realist evaluation of nursing practice

In England, Jeffries et al. (2017) conducted a realist evaluation to examine the implementation of a new electronic system for optimising a drug administration system into a general practice context. They conducted five semi-structured interviews, four focus groups and one observation with key stakeholders. The researchers found that the system improved patient safety outcomes and there was better identification of patients who were at risk of developing adverse drug events. However, they also concluded that effective use depended on how engaged health professionals were with the system and the information flow between the different professionals.

M. Jeffries, D.I. Phipps, R.L. Howards, A.J. Avery, S. Rodgers & D.M. Ashcroft, 2017, 'Understanding the implementation and adoption of a technological intervention to improve medication safety in primary care: A realist evaluation', *BMC Health Services Research*, vol. 17, article 196.

Questions for consideration
- Why was realist evaluation an appropriate design for this study?
- How might the findings lead to enhanced care delivery?

RESEARCH EXAMPLE 8.4 Realist evaluation of midwifery practice

In Scotland, Doi et al. (2015) conducted a realist evaluation of screening and a brief alcohol intervention program in routine antenatal care at two maternity hospitals. They used a three-phase approach:

1 The researchers identified the program theory. They interviewed four stakeholders involved in policy implementation and conducted a systematic review.

2 The researchers tested the program, conducting interviews with seventeen pregnant women and fifteen midwives, and a focus group with six midwifery team leaders.

3 Through data analysis and interpretation, the researchers refined the program theory.

The researchers found that the program elicited positive attitudes towards alcohol consumption during pregnancy, but the small number of participants meant the program was not necessarily delivered as anticipated. They identified important contextual aspects in the woman–midwife relationship and challenges in negotiating the timing of screening and delivery of the intervention.

L. Doi, R. Jepson & H. Cheyne, 2015, 'A realist evaluation of an antenatal programme to change drinking behaviour of pregnant women', *Midwifery*, vol. 31, pp. 965–972.

Questions for consideration
- Why was realist evaluation an appropriate design for this study?
- How might the findings lead to enhanced care delivery?

CHAPTER SUMMARY

Nurses and midwives need to have the knowledge and skills to implement new knowledge into practice, to ensure they deliver best practice. Successful implementation of evidence-based practice requires a systematic and well-informed approach. This chapter has introduced the concept of knowledge translation and processes for questioning current practices. It has examined places for sourcing quality evidence, and processes and structures that can be employed to successfully implement new evidence into practice.

CHAPTER REVIEW QUESTIONS

- Why is implementation of new evidence into nursing and midwifery practice important?
- Who is responsible for implementing new evidence into practice?
- Why is evaluation of implementation of new practice needed?
- How can approaches such as action research and realist evaluation assist with evaluating practice change?

QUESTIONS FOR DISCUSSION

- What might be facilitators and barriers to the implementation of new evidence into clinical nursing or midwifery practice?
- What strategies could be used to manage these?

QUESTIONS FOR PERSONAL REFLECTION

- How much do you consider evidence in your own practice?
- What might assist you to be more focused on evidence in your practice?

USEFUL WEB RESOURCES

Australian Nursing and Midwifery Federation's nursing and midwifery research policy
<http://anmf.org.au/documents/policies/P_Nursing_Midwifery_Research.pdf>
Johns Hopkins Medicine's Johns Hopkins Nursing Evidence-Based Practice Model
<www.hopkinsmedicine.org/evidence-based-practice/ijhn_2017_ebp.html>
National Health and Medical Research Council's Australian clinical practice guidelines
<www.clinicalguidelines.gov.au>
National Institute for Health and Care Excellence (United Kingdom) <www.nice.org.uk>

REFERENCES AND FURTHER READING

Benjamin, A., 2008, 'Audit: How to do it in practice', *British Medical Journal*, vol. 336, 1241–1245.

Casey, M., O'Leary, D. & Coghlan, D., 2017, 'Unpacking action research and implementation science: Implications for nursing', *Journal of Advanced Nursing*, doi: 10.1111/jan.13494.

Doi, L., Jepson, R. & Cheyne, H., 2015, 'A realist evaluation of an antenatal programme to change drinking behaviour of pregnant women', *Midwifery*, vol. 31, pp. 965–972.

Eccles, M.P. & Mittman, B.S. 2006, 'Welcome to Implementation Science', *Implementation Science*, doi.org/10.1186/1748-5908-1-1.

Fairbrother, G., Cashin, A., Conway, R. & Graham, I., 2016, 'Evidence based nursing and midwifery practice in a regional Australian healthcare setting: Behaviours, skills and barriers', *Collegian*, vol. 23, pp. 29–37.

Flynn, M. & Quinn, J., 2010, 'Research dissemination and knowledge translation', *British Journal of Cardiac Nursing*, vol. 5, no. 12, pp. 600–604.

Friesen-Storms, J.H.H.M., Moser, A., van der Loo, S., Beurskens, A.J.H.M. & Bours, G.J.J.W., 2014, 'Systematic implementation of evidence-based practice in a clinical nursing setting: A participatory action research project', *Journal of Clinical Nursing*, vol. 24, pp. 57–68.

Hegney D. & Francis K., 2015, 'Action research: Changing nursing practice', *Nursing Standard*, vol. 29, no. 40, pp. 36–41.

Jeffries, M., Phipps, D.L., Howards, R.L., Avery, A.J., Rodgers, S. & Ashcroft, D.M., 2017, 'Understanding the implementation and adoption of a technological intervention to improve medication safety in primary care: A realist evaluation', *BMC Health Services Research*, vol. 17, article 196.

Johns Hopkins Medicine, 2017, *Johns Hopkins Nursing Evidence-Based Practice Model*, <www.hopkinsmedicine.org/evidence-based-practice/ijhn_2017_ebp.html>.

Kitson, A.L., Harvey, G. & McCormack, B., 1998, 'Enabling the implementation of evidence based practice: A conceptual framework', *Quality in Health Care*, vol. 7, pp. 149–158.

Kitson, A.L. & Harvey, G., 2016, 'Methods to succeed in effective knowledge translation in clinical practice', *Journal of Nursing Scholarship*, vol. 48, no. 3, pp. 294–302.

Leeman, J. & Sandelowski, M., 2012, 'Practice-based evidence and qualitative inquiry', *Journal of Nursing Scholarship*, vol. 44, no. 2, pp. 171–179.

Melnyk, B.M. & Fineout-Overholt, E., 2010, 'ARCC (Advancing Research and Clinical Practice through Close Collaboration): A model for system-wide implementation and sustainability of evidence-based practice', in J. Rycroft-Malone & T. Bucknall (eds), *Models and Frameworks for Implementing Evidence-Based Practice: Linking evidence to action*, West Sussex: Wiley-Blackwell, pp. 169–184.

Munten, G., van den Bogaard, J., Cox, K., Garretson, H. & Bongers, I., 2010, 'Implementation of evidence-based practice in nursing using action research: A review', *Worldviews on Evidence-Based Nursing*, vol. 7, no. 3, pp. 135–157.

Nairn, S., 'A critical realist approach to knowledge: Implications for evidence-based practice in and beyond nursing', *Nursing Inquiry*, vol. 19, no. 1, pp. 6–17.

National Health and Medical Research Council *see* NHMRC

NHMRC, 2017, *Clinical Practice Guidelines Portal*, <www.clinicalguidelines.gov.au/portal>.

Nilson, P., 2015, 'Making sense of implementation theories, models and frameworks', *Implementation Science*, doi.org/10.1186/s13012-015-0242-0.

Pawson, R. & Tilley, N., 1997, *Realistic Evaluation*, London: Sage.

Pawson, R. & Tilley, N., 2004, *Realist Evaluation*, Community Matters, <www.communitymatters.com.au/RE_chapter.pdf>.

Quinn, E., Noble, J., Seale, H. & Ward, J.E., 2013, 'Investigating the potential for evidence-based midwifery-led services in very remote Australia: Viewpoints from local stakeholders', *Women and Birth*, vol. 26, pp. 254–259.

Rowles, E. & McNaughton, A., 2017, 'An overview of the evidence-based practice process for novice researchers', *Nursing Standard*, vol. 31, no. 43, pp. 50–60.

Spruce, L., 2015, 'Back to basics: Implementing evidence-based practice', *AORN Journal*, vol. 101, no. 1, pp. 107–112.

Tiller, M., 2007, 'Translating research into practice', *American Journal of Nursing*, vol. 107, no. 6 supp., pp. 26–33.

Van Achterberg, T., 2013, 'Nursing implementation science: 10 ways forward', *International Journal of Nursing Studies*, vol. 50, pp. 445–447.

Wallin, L., 2008, 'Knowledge translation and implementation research in nursing', *International Journal of Nursing Studies*, vol. 46, pp. 576–587.

Yoder, L.H., Kirkley, D., McFall, D.C., Kirksey, K.M., StalBaum, A.L. & Sellers, D., 2014, 'Staff nurses' use of research to facilitate evidence-based practice', *American Journal of Nursing*, vol. 114, no. 9, pp. 26–37.

CHAPTER 9

Writing effective reviews of literature

LEARNING OBJECTIVES

After working through this chapter, you should be able to:

- discuss why literature reviews are important for evidence-based nursing and midwifery practice
- identify different types of literature reviews
- outline the key reasons for performing a literature review
- identify steps involved in developing a quality literature review
- plan and write a quality literature review.

KEY TERMS AND CONCEPTS

Direct quotation, grey literature, literature review, paraphrasing, primary source, secondary source, synthesis

CASE STUDY OVERVIEW

April is a first-year student who has been given the following assignment for her clinical subject, in which medication management has just been introduced: 'With reference to the literature, critically explore issues around medication administration by nurses and midwives'. April recognises that to do this, she needs to do a literature review. She has never written a formal review before and does not really know how to go about it.

CHAPTER INTRODUCTION

In Chapter 6, we explored different types of literature reviews commonly used in nursing and midwifery—namely, the traditional narrative review, systematic review and scoping review. We also explored the processes for searching for literature and critically appraising it. This chapter builds on that content to examine the process of making sense of the research literature and putting it together in a meaningful and quality review that can form a basis on which to deliver evidence-based practice.

What is a literature review?

A **literature review** is 'a comprehensive overview of prior research regarding a specific topic' (Denney & Tewksbury 2012, p. 218). A sound literature review provides an overview of the key ideas around what is known on the topic of interest. In addition, it identifies where there are gaps in what is known on the topic and where future research might be warranted.

literature review
a synthesis of previously published research conducted on a particular topic

Literature reviews are common academic assessment tasks. However, the skills needed for conducting and writing them are also important for nursing and midwifery practice. Clinical guidelines to inform practice should be developed after rigorous reviews of previous studies have ensured that all appropriate evidence on which to base that practice has been appraised and synthesised. The ability to communicate findings of such a review is also therefore paramount to the development of strong clinical guidelines (Fowler 2014). According to Baker (2016), literature reviews serve a number of purposes:

- They provide a sound framework for presenting knowledge of a particular topic.
- They identify and define the key terms and important variables used in the existing studies.
- They provide new perspectives and a collated overview of current evidence to support practice, and they challenge assumptions and opinions.

- They identify the main research approaches used by previous researchers exploring the particular topic.
- They demonstrate where there might be gaps in current knowledge for which new research could be devised.

Types of literature reviews

There are many types of literature reviews. They can be descriptive or traditional in nature, such as narrative review, purely describing the available literature, or they can take a very structured approach, such as in a systematic or scoping review. According to Denney and Tewksbury (2012, p. 4), the focus of a literature review can be 'integrative (summarizing past research based on overall conclusions of the past research), theoretical (identifying and critiquing the ability of different theories to explain a phenomenon), or methodological (highlighting different methodological approaches used in past research and the contributions of each type of research)'.

ACTIVITY 9.1 Types of literature reviews

- Review the types of literature reviews presented in Chapter 6.
- Summarise the key differences between them.

RESEARCH EXAMPLE 9.1 Narrative review of medication administration error

Medication administration is a key component of the nurse's role. Errors in medication administration pose major risks to patient safety, so understanding causes of errors is important for practice. Parry et al. (2015) conducted a narrative review to explore factors contributing to registered nurses' behaviours around medication administration. They included 26 papers dating from 1999 to 2012 and originating predominantly from North America and Europe. They presented their analysis in two domains: *environment* and *person*. In the environment domain, aspects like clinical workload, patient acuity, interruptions, teamwork, communication and organisation work were found to be contributing factors. In the person domain, reported characteristics impacting on the registered nurses' work included fatigue, shift patterns and quality of work life. The researchers recommended a shift in thinking, from errors being seen as events to being viewed as the interplay between the person, environment and medication administration behaviour.

A.M. Parry, K.L. Barriball & A.E. While, 2015, 'Factors contributing to registered nurse medication administration error: A narrative review', *International Journal of Nursing Studies*, vol. 52, pp. 403–420.

Questions for consideration
- How could the findings from this narrative review help to guide medication administration practice?
- How could collating research findings from a number of studies like this assist us to better understand the area of medication administration?

Writing a literature review

Clarifying the question

Before embarking on a literature review, it is important to understand what is required of the review. If it is for an academic assignment and the topic is provided, it is crucial to carefully consider what is being asked and what the keywords are in the question. If the topic has to be determined, consider a question that is not too broad and can be easily managed. You can get a sense of how much literature is available on a topic by doing a quick database search. If the topic appears to have been very well researched, narrow the focus to something more manageable. It will be much easier to move on to the detailed search if the question is well crafted beforehand. University and hospital librarians can be of great assistance in helping to refine literature searches, so it may be useful to seek one out at this point.

Searching for literature

In Chapters 2 and 6, we touched on searching for literature and quality appraisal of research. Before you can undertake a review, you need to determine the keywords that you are going to use to search for relevant literature. These will be directly related to your research question or topic but you need to consider variations, such as synonyms, for each word to ensure the review is broad enough. To do this effectively takes time, but it will enhance the quality of the review. As identified in Chapter 2, the US National Library of Medicine (2018) has a very useful website of Medical Subject Headings, where you can search for additional keywords and extend the literature search to ensure as many articles as possible are captured.

At this point, it is also important to consider what you will include in your review. It is common practice to decide on a date range from which literature will be sourced. If you are performing a review of research for current practice, it is not sensible to draw recommendations from outdated research. As a rule of thumb, literature should be no more than ten years old. However, for some clinical practices or academic requirements much more recent literature might be required, particularly if the aim is to identify gaps in current knowledge. On the other hand, you may need to go further back than ten years when knowledge is well established and does not need to be researched again. It is important also to decide whether only research studies—quantitative, qualitative or both—will be included in the review or whether other types of materials, such as reports, clinical guidelines and discussion papers, will be included, and why.

Literature for review can be accessed from a number of sources. However, it is necessary to check the quality of the material you source and only use that which you can clearly see is credible. Most resources are likely to come from databases accessed through your university or hospital library. In addition to material sourced through databases, you can also seek out grey literature, for example, reports or clinical guidelines available from other sources, such as professional and government organisations. The search engine Google Scholar can be particularly useful in searching for other types of credible materials that might not be listed on databases.

There are some important tricks in searching for appropriate research literature. One of these is using truncations—that is, parts of words that may appear in different forms. This concept was introduced in Chapter 2, so you may wish to review that chapter before you continue on.

ACTIVITY 9.2 Searching for literature

In this chapter's case study, first-year student April has to do a literature review for one of her assessment tasks. She has been asked to use literature to critically explore issues around medication administration by nurses and midwives.

1 Develop a list of keywords that April could use to search for relevant literature.
2 Using these keywords, go to one of the databases in Research Tip 2.1 that you have not used before and conduct a search. Try including some Boolean operators and truncators in the format for that database.
3 List the challenges you encounter.
4 Search on Google Scholar for literature that may assist April.

Questions for consideration

• What differences do you note between the relevance and specificity of hits from the database and the search engine?
• How might these differences impact on the way you use each?

Selecting literature to include

Generally, a search of databases will yield many more articles than you need for a review. However, many may also be irrelevant to the topic you are exploring, or they may not meet your initial inclusion criteria. In Chapter 6, we examined the process of determining the scope of systematic and scoping reviews. Sometimes, these approaches can also be useful in facilitating more focused narrative reviews. In addition, the tools covered in that chapter provide a foundation for determining the quality of the research evidence and could be used to assist with deciding what to include in a more general review.

Reading and critiquing the literature

Careful reading and re-reading of each sourced paper is needed to fully grasp the main concepts presented in it. As you do this, it is important to write in your own words notes of your interpretations of the key aspects. This helps to ensure you have fully understood the paper and the author's discussion. Begin to group papers into those with similar focuses. This will assist you when it comes to planning out the review. Remember to note down the relevant details required for referencing the paper, to make the process of writing the report smoother.

Consider also the nature of the material. Papers that you use in your review should be **primary sources**; that is, the research should be directly reported by the researchers who actually conducted the research study. **Secondary sources** are those where the authors are reporting on someone else's research, so they provide a second-hand account of the work. In this case, they may not give an accurate description of the actual research study. If you notice you have a secondary reference, it is best to seek out the original or to not make use of the work in your review. Textbooks are usually considered secondary references, unless they are providing first-hand reports of research written by the researchers who conducted the study.

primary source
a paper that provides first-hand reporting of a study by the researcher

secondary source
a paper that reports on someone else's research study

Synthesising ideas and planning the review

Just like planning for any essay, a written plan is important for ensuring that a clear line of argument and flow of ideas appears in the final review. This should include an introduction, body and conclusion. For a high-quality review, careful planning of ideas and their flow is needed.

Introduction

The review will begin with an introduction. This establishes and explains the argument that the paper is making, defines any keywords or terminology and provides necessary background to the topic. It gives the reader an idea of the direction that the review will take.

Review body

The body of the literature review provides the main discussion and argument. From your reading and summarising, you will have ascertained the key ideas and concepts to be covered. These will become the topic sentences presenting the key messages that will subsequently form each of the paragraphs. It is important to organise these ideas in such a way that the overall content and argument flow logically from the beginning to the end of the work. Thus, the ideas covered in each paragraph should build on those in the previous paragraph and lead into those in the next.

Conclusion

The conclusion draws together the key ideas presented in the work. It might also include discussion of limitations in the existing body of literature and make recommendations for future research.

Writing the review

Once you have developed the plan for your literature review, you can begin to write. As you do this, you will need to present the ideas from the research papers you have read and summarised. However, the review should not just read like a list of quotations or jump from idea to idea without a clear flow. The reader should be led from a very broad, general introduction of the topic to a specific focus. It needs to be clear that you have synthesised and carefully considered the ideas of different authors and are not just reporting their findings one after the other. Remember that you need to create a consistent line of argument that flows throughout the work. Your plan should have been developed in such a way as to allow you to create meaningful paragraphs that fit together seamlessly. Any claims made or conclusions presented in the review need to be supported by appropriate research evidence.

Paraphrasing is an important strategy in academic writing. This involves rewriting key ideas in your own words. Many people make the mistake of merely replacing a few words throughout a piece of text and believing they have paraphrased. This is not considered to be paraphrasing; rather the material needs to be rewritten in other words but retaining the concept, argument or

paraphrasing
rewriting ideas in one's own words

idea that the original author was making. Whenever you are presenting the ideas of another author or researcher—that is, not your own original thoughts—you must also cite the person (or people) who originally documented them.

ACTIVITY 9.3 Paraphrasing

1 Source the full text of one of the research articles on medication administration issues that you located for Activity 9.2.
2 Select one or two paragraphs and paraphrase the key points that the author is making in them.
3 Note down your experiences of doing this.

Question for consideration

• What things did you need to be mindful of?

You can also use **direct quotation**s to support arguments—that is, word-for-word text from a research paper. However, it is a good idea to keep these to a minimum where possible, for use when a concept is too difficult to paraphrase or with ideas that are fundamental to the research. Present direct quotations clearly, in quotation marks, indicating that the work is that of another author. Many referencing style approaches, for example, APA or Harvard, will also require you to add the page number of the original source.

direct quotation
text taken word-for-word from another person's work; this requires the inclusion of quotation marks, citation and possibly also the page number of the work from which the words were taken

The word length of a quotation will determine where in the text it is placed. Depending on the referencing style used, quotes longer than 30 to 40 words may start on a new line and be indented. If your literature review has a prescribed word count, remember that quotations generally do not contribute to it, as they do not constitute your own words.

The way your work will be interpreted by an independent reader needs careful consideration as you write. While you will likely know all of the studies covered in your review very well, the reader may not. You need to provide enough detail of each study for the reader to understand the context and the argument that you are making. In our case study, for example, April could write in her review, 'Choo et al. (2013) found that nurses were distracted during medication administration'. However, the reader would understand much more of the context of the study if April wrote this as 'Choo et al. (2013) found using observation that nurses in two hospitals in Singapore were distracted by other personnel and telephone calls during medication administration'.

It is important to present a balanced perspective. Not all research that you include will necessarily support your original assumptions. Noting differences in study designs and outcomes, and conflicting findings as well as similar findings, should form part of the picture. Keep in mind that while you may have a particular belief about the topic, very different findings may emerge from the literature. The review should not reflect your personal beliefs; rather, it must reflect what is actually presented through the literature.

RESEARCH EXAMPLE 9.2 Systematic review of medication administration error and near-miss reporting

Medication administration forms a large part of the nurse's role, and errors pose a major risk to patient safety. However, the scope of medication errors and near misses may not be fully reported. Vrbnjak et al. (2016) conducted a systematic review to explore the barriers to nurses reporting medication errors and near misses in hospital environments. They found 38 articles that met their inclusion criteria. The researchers grouped their findings into two categories: *organisational barriers* and *personal/ professional barriers*. Organisational barriers included the workplace culture, types of systems in place for reporting and behaviours of managers—for example, focusing on the individual and not the system. Personal/professional barriers included fear of blame and stigmatisation, not taking responsibility for the outcome, denial, and lack of education or knowledge about what and how to report. The researchers recommended that there needed to be a sense of trust between nurses and their managers, reporting systems that were not complicated and time consuming, recognition that most errors were the result of the system and not the individual, and ongoing education and training about reporting all errors and near misses.

D. Vrbnjak, S. Denieffe, C. O'Gorman & M. Pajnkihar, 2016, 'Barriers to reporting medication errors and near misses among nurses: A systematic review', *International Journal of Nursing Studies*, vol. 63, pp. 162–178.

Questions for consideration

- How could findings from this systematic review help to broadly inform evidence-based medication administration practice?
- What value can reviews of literature have for other areas of clinical practice?

ACTIVITY 9.4 Approaching a literature review

In our case study, April has been asked to undertake a literature review on issues around medication administration by nurses and midwives. She has never written a formal review before and comes to you for advice. Using the knowledge you have gained in this chapter, summarise the information she needs to successfully complete the assessment.

CHAPTER SUMMARY

Literature reviews can provide valuable information with which to inform evidence-based nursing and midwifery practice. This chapter has examined practicalities in performing reviews of the research literature. The importance of refining the research question, carefully developing and managing the search, and planning and writing the review has been examined.

CHAPTER REVIEW QUESTIONS

- Why is it important for nurses and midwives to be able to write quality literature reviews?
- What are the key aspects to consider in selecting research literature to include in a review?
- What are important factors to consider in writing a literature review?

QUESTIONS FOR DISCUSSION

- How can we utilise literature reviews to enhance evidence-based practice?
- What are the key skills needed to produce high-quality literature reviews?
- What might be limitations to the use of literature reviews to inform evidence-based practice?

QUESTIONS FOR PERSONAL REFLECTION

- How have you approached writing literature reviews in the past?
- How might you now do that differently?

USEFUL WEB RESOURCES

Australian Nursing and Midwifery Federation's nursing and midwifery research policy
<http://anmf.org.au/documents/policies/P_Nursing_Midwifery_Research.pdf>
US National Library of Medicine's Medical Subject Headings <www.nlm.nih.gov/mesh/>

REFERENCES AND FURTHER READING

Baker, J.D., 2016, 'The purpose, process, and methods of writing a literature review', *AORN Journal*, vol. 103, no. 3, pp. 265–269.

Burden, B., 2001, 'Writing a review of the literature: A practical guide', *British Journal of Midwifery*, vol. 9, no. 8, pp. 498–501.

Choo, J., Johnston, L. & Manias, E., 2013, 'Nurses' medication administration practices at two Singaporean acute care hospitals', *Nursing and Health Sciences*, vol. 15, pp. 101–108.

Cronin, P., Ryan, F. & Coughlan, M., 2008, 'Undertaking a literature review: A step-by-step approach', *British Journal of Nursing*, vol. 17, no. 1, pp. 38–43.

Denney, A.S. & Tewksbury, R., 2012, 'How to write a literature review', *Journal of Criminal Justice Education*, vol. 24, no. 2, pp. 218–234.

Fowler, J., 2014, 'Written communication: From staff nurse to nurse consultant', part 5: 'Literature reviews', *British Journal of Nursing*, vol. 23, no. 19, p. 1046.

Galdas, P., 2014, 'Searching for the evidence', *Nursing Standard*, vol. 28, no. 40, p. 66.

Haddaway, N.R., Collins, A.M., Coughlin, D. & Kirk, S., 2015, 'The role of Google Scholar in evidence reviews and its applicability to grey literature searching', *PLOS One*, vol. 10, no. 9, e0138237, doi: 10.1371/journal.pone.0138237.

Jaidka, K., Khoo, C.S.G. & Na, J.-C., 2013, 'Literature review writing: How information is selected and transformed', *Aslib Proceedings: New Information Perspectives*, vol. 65, no. 3, pp. 303–325.

Lingard, L., 2017, 'Writing an effective literature review', *Perspectives on Medical Education*, vol. 7, pp. 47–49.

Parry, A.M., Barriball, K.L. & While, A.E., 2015, 'Factors contributing to registered nurse medication administration error: A narrative review', *International Journal of Nursing Studies*, vol. 52, pp. 403–420.

Pautasso, M., 2013, 'Ten simple rules for writing a literature review', *PLOS Computational Biology*, vol. 9, no. 7, e10033149, doi: 10.1371/journal.pcbi.1003149.

US National Library of Medicine, 2018, *Medical Subject Headings*, <www.nlm.nih.gov/mesh/>.

Vrbnjak, D., Denieffe, S., O'Gorman, C. & Pajnkihar, M., 2016, 'Barriers to reporting medication errors and near misses among nurses: A systematic review', *International Journal of Nursing Studies*, vol. 63, pp. 162–178.

Wakefield, A., 2014, 'Searching and critiquing the research literature', *Nursing Standard*, vol. 28, no. 39, pp. 49–57.

Winchester, C.L. & Salji, M., 2016, 'Writing a literature review', *Journal of Clinical Urology*, vol. 9, no. 5, pp. 308–312.

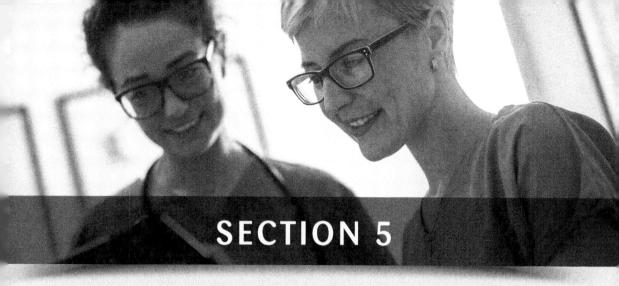

SECTION 5

HOW DO I PURSUE A NURSING OR MIDWIFERY RESEARCH FUTURE?

So far in this book, we have focused on understanding research and its application to nursing and midwifery through evidence-based practice. However, increasingly, nurses and midwives are driving research projects and the generation of quality knowledge to support practice. Many do this as part of their clinical or academic roles, while others seek to pursue a purely research-focused role, specialising in the generation of new knowledge. So, while you may be thinking about what type of clinical role you would like to focus on in your future career, research is a pathway. This section, consisting of one final chapter, introduces various options for research careers in nursing and midwifery. It examines different educational pathways to research careers, whether these be clinically or academically focused.

Increasingly, nurses and midwives are seeking ways to attract funding, small and large, to support their research activity. This might be for a small research project in a single ward area or a large, multi-centre clinical trial. The skill of writing research proposals is important to success. Some undergraduate and postgraduate courses include the writing of research proposals, so in the second part of this section, we present a step-by-step approach to developing your own quality research proposal.

CHAPTER 10

Research pathways for nurses and midwives

LEARNING OBJECTIVES

After working through this chapter, you should be able to:

- define the term *clinical trial*
- identify research roles that nurses and midwives can undertake
- discuss the role played by the research nurse or research midwife
- identify research pathways for nurses and midwives
- explore opportunities for seeking funding for research ideas
- identify the key components of a research proposal
- write a quality research proposal.

KEY TERMS AND CONCEPTS

Clinical doctorate, clinical trial nurse, evidence generator, funding, midwife researcher, nurse researcher, research degree, research midwife, research nurse, research proposal

CASE STUDY OVERVIEW

Angela is a clinical nurse specialist working in a busy women's health unit. She is really interested in getting involved in research, having completed a masters degree and undertaken a small research project as part of her studies. An opportunity has arisen for Angela to take on a role as a clinical research nurse in a new funded project being undertaken by a group of researchers exploring the effectiveness of a newly available drug for managing the effects of early menopause. She decides that this is a great opportunity to develop her research skills so agrees to take up the role.

CHAPTER INTRODUCTION

Research plays an important role in the everyday lives of all nurses and midwives in the delivery of effective and evidence-based care. However, the use and conduct of research in nursing and midwifery can be much broader than merely implementing the findings of others into practice. While many nurses choose to specialise within the vast array of clinical specialty areas, there are many ways in which nurses and midwives can also be active in the generation of research and even specialise in research roles. Some of these are clinically based, while others are more distant from the bedside. In this chapter, we will explore research roles in the two disciplines, including the possible pathways to a research career.

Increasingly, there is an expectation that midwives and nurses in clinical practice roles will engage with research findings, to underpin their practice, as well as in the generation of research studies. Sometimes, there are opportunities to apply for funding to support engagement in research activities, so skills in writing funding proposals are important. In the second half of the chapter, we will explore the fundamental aspects of developing a research proposal, either for the purposes of further studies or for attracting funding to support research activities.

Evidence generator: The nurse/midwife as researcher

Throughout this text, we have introduced basic concepts underpinning research, including approaches to doing research and to critiquing and utilising the research conducted by others. However, increasingly, there are specific research roles for nurses and midwives, particularly in clinical settings. These offer unique opportunities for individuals interested in pursuing research careers, including for the **research nurse** or **research midwife**, nurse or midwife researcher and academic researcher.

research nurse
a nurse who works with a team on a clinical trial

research midwife
a midwife who works with a team on a clinical trial

Research nurse or midwife

Research roles for nurses and midwives are growing. A role that is not well written about is that of the research nurse or midwife. Also known as *clinical research nurses, clinical trial nurses* or *clinical research midwives*, they play an important role in managing funded research projects, specifically

clinical trials—that is, studies that seek to examine the effectiveness of new treatments in clinical practice with a view to enhancing or changing the management of patients. Research nurses and midwives are employed in research-specific locations or on research projects for the duration of the funded study.

clinical trial
a study that examines the effectiveness of new treatments in clinical practice with a view to enhancing or changing the management of patients

Globally, numbers of clinical trials are growing, and, thus, the demand for research nurses—and, to a lesser extent, research midwives—has grown. Clinical trials are common for testing new medications, medical devices or changes in usual approaches to care. To ensure they are of the highest quality, clinical trials are conducted in a very rigorous way and often involve a number of professionals, such as doctors, nurses, midwives, pharmacists and allied health professionals (Bowrey & Thompson 2014).

Research nurses and midwives undertake a variety of roles. Traditionally, these have been very limited, such as collecting samples, in the actual research process. However, the roles have expanded significantly, and the following activities are now commonly undertaken by research nurses and midwives:

- managing projects from beginning to end
- recruiting participants, usually patients or other healthcare consumers
- communicating with other health professionals, project team members and relevant authorities related to the study
- managing data collection, which might include taking samples (for example, blood or urine) or monitoring (for example, blood pressure)
- entering data into computer programs or project paperwork
- contributing to the development of new treatments (for example, new medications)
- working within a multidisciplinary team that may include doctors, pharmacists, allied health professionals and scientists
- interacting with patient participants, including coordinating appointments and clinical procedures
- monitoring the effects of interventions (for example, new treatments)
- identifying and reporting adverse events
- ensuring the safety of participants

- ensuring the study adheres to study protocols and ethical and legislative requirements
- submitting project reports
- promoting research awareness and research culture among key stakeholders.

In the United Kingdom, Kunhunny and Salmon (2017) undertook a study to explore the professional identity of the clinical research nurse. They interviewed eleven clinical research nurses about their roles and professional identities. The findings indicated that the nurses were very satisfied with their ability to act as 'agents of change in health care' through their research engagement.

ACTIVITY 10.1 Exploring the clinical research nurse role

In this chapter's case study, Angela has agreed to take on a clinical research nurse role in a project exploring the effectiveness of a new drug for managing the effects of early menopause. List the types of activities Angela may be required to undertake as part of this role.

RESEARCH EXAMPLE 10.1 Clinical trial nurses in Australia

The number of clinical trials conducted around the world is growing, and this has generated increasing demand for clinical research nurses, or clinical trial nurses. Wilkes et al. (2012) undertook a study using survey methodology to explore the roles of clinical trial nurses in Australia. They found that there was a range of terms used to describe the role, including *clinical trials coordinator* (the most prevalent), *clinical research coordinator, clinical research nurse, clinical research manager, research associate* and *research midwife*. They reported that 86.6 per cent had no formal research training. Despite the integral nature of their roles, more than half reported not being cited as co-authors of research publications. The researchers found there were differences in the roles that clinical trial nurses performed. Some performed primarily day-to-day operational roles (such as managing data, ensuring informed consent was received from participants and recruitment), while others played higher order roles (such as protocol or study planning).

L. Wilkes, D. Jackson, C. Miranda & R. Watson, 2012, 'The role of clinical trial nurses: An Australian perspective', *Collegian*, vol. 19, pp. 239–246.

Questions for consideration

- What are some of the issues associated with the clinical trial nurse's role as reported in the study?
- How should the role develop in the future?

Nurse or midwife researcher

There are a number of models by which **nurse researchers** and **midwife researchers** may work in research. Often, they work in academic or clinical settings, or both, on studies focused on issues or care aspects that particularly concern nursing or midwifery. Hence, they usually contribute knowledge to the nursing or midwifery disciplines. It is common for nurse or midwife researchers to design and conduct their own projects (Watmough et al. 2010), as opposed to working in a clinical research team. These research roles can be combined with an academic teaching role or can be standalone research positions.

nurse researcher
a nurse who conducts research

midwife researcher
a midwife who conducts research

Education pathways to research roles in nursing and midwifery

Growing recognition of the role of nurses and midwives in research-related activity has led to a growth in the need for higher level education and research preparation. While at an undergraduate level, students learn about the role of research, types of studies and how to interpret research, higher degree courses give nurses and midwives the opportunity to develop skills in doing research, so that they can become researchers, in clinical, academic or other settings, and contribute to the nursing knowledge base. While there are a variety, all higher degree courses, or **research degrees**, require students to undertake some research. People are often fearful of this, as they feel unprepared to carry out their own research. However, it is important to recognise that all of these pathways are designed to provide research training—that is, learning to do research. If you choose to take up such an option, you are not expected to work alone but will have the support and guidance of an academic mentor who will work with you throughout the study.

research degree
a degree that entails conducting a research study

honours degree
an undergraduate research degree, usually comprising one year of full-time-equivalent study

Honours degrees

An honours degree is an undergraduate award offered by many universities to highly achieving students. It is the equivalent of one academic year and commonly provides students with grounding in research methods and the opportunity to complete a small-scale research study under the supervision of academic staff. Honours degrees can provide direct entry into doctoral studies if the grades achieved meet individual university entrance requirements. Sometimes, honours degrees are integrated into graduate nurse or midwife programs.

RESEARCH EXAMPLE 10.2 Honours degrees in Australia

Honours degrees have been offered in Australia for many years as pathways to postgraduate, or higher degree, studies. Traditionally, they involve carrying out a small research study and submission of a thesis or report. Halcomb et al. (2018) conducted a survey of coordinators of nursing honours programs across Australia. Fifteen respondents reported on their honours programs. The researchers identified variety in the types of programs offered and in the assessment requirements. They also found that there was a perception that honours degrees were not often valued in clinical practice. However, they stressed that the value in honours degrees is their potential to steer students towards leadership roles in nursing, as well as towards doctoral studies.

E. Halcomb, E. Smyth, L. Moxham, V. Traynor & R. Fernandez, 2018, 'Bachelor of nursing programs in Australia: Trends and key challenges', *Collegian*, doi: 10.1016/j. colegn.2017.11.003.

Questions for consideration

- What are some of the issues associated with honours degrees?
- What factors would impact on your consideration of studying for an honours degree?
- How could honours degrees benefit clinical practice?

Masters degrees

Most universities offering nursing or midwifery courses also offer masters degrees. There is a variety of these on offer; some consist of all course-work, others offer coursework as well as a small-scale research study, and others can be done purely by conducting and reporting on a research study. Coursework components can be generic or pathways to specialised practice, such as intensive care or emergency nursing. Students doing coursework masters degrees who also have the opportunity to undertake a research study should seriously consider doing so, as it may later provide entry pathways into doctoral studies, and it is wise to keep future employment and study options open.

Doctor of Philosophy

The Doctor of Philosophy (or PhD) is a postgraduate degree entirely consisting of a large research study and is the usual pathway for an individual seeking an academic career in a university or as a full-time researcher. At the end of the course, the candidate is required to submit for examination a thesis, usually around 80,000 to 100,000 words in length. The impetus for research conducted at doctoral level may be a study devised by the student, or the research may form part of a larger study managed by the supervisor.

Professional doctorates

Professional doctorates are gaining popularity in clinical disciplines like nursing and midwifery, where they are often known as **clinical doctorates** and may also be titled *Doctor of Nursing, Doctor of Nursing Practice* or *Doctor of Midwifery*. They were originally introduced to provide entry to advanced practice in health disciplines such as pharmacy and physiotherapy (Cronenwett et al. 2011) and aim largely to develop research skills in clinicians wanting to deliver evidence-based care. In clinical areas, they are highly valued over the Doctor of Philosophy, which is seen to be more removed from the clinical setting. Professional doctorates focus on research that can be translated directly into practice, making a change at the point of care (Florczak et al. 2014). They usually consist of some coursework followed by the conduct of a supervised clinical research study and submission of a thesis, usually around 60,000 words in length.

clinical doctorate
a clinically focused doctoral degree

ACTIVITY 10.2 Exploring a research career

In our case study, Angela was employed as a research nurse. The funded research project is coming to an end, and she is considering her future professional role. She has enjoyed the research role and decides that she wants to pursue a research career.

Questions for consideration
- What options does she have for moving in that direction?
- What educational programs could Angela undertake to support her moving into a research career?

Seeking funding for clinical research

One challenge faced by researchers is that of funding their research activity. Funding is used to support the costs of the study, including research assistant salaries, materials for collecting specimens, professional transcription of interview transcripts, and equipment, such as computer

ACTIVITY 10.3 Personal reflection

Think about your future direction in nursing or midwifery.

Questions for consideration
- Where do you see yourself working in the next five years?
- How might a research degree help you along that pathway?
- What type of research degree should you be considering given that direction? Why?

software and audio-recorders. Fortunately, much of the research undertaken by nurses and midwives does not require extensive funding. Yet, having funding can be the deciding factor in whether a study proceeds or not. Funding can be difficult to source, and funding applications are usually part of a competitive process. There are several options for researchers seeking funding:

- National research organisations (for example, the Australian Research Council and the National Health and Medical Research Council) provide large-scale competitive funding for research conducted by experienced researchers.
- There are many professional nursing and midwifery organisations (for example, the Australian College of Nursing, the Australian College of Midwives and the Australian Nursing and Midwifery Federation) that provide funding that is often sufficient for small projects conducted by nurses and midwives.
- Specific medical support organisations often have funding rounds to support research related to the condition on which they focus.
- Often, healthcare organisations offer internal funding—small research grants—to support clinicians to undertake research in their clinical areas.
- There are competitive opportunities for researchers to develop their research skills through fellowships that provide supporting salaries for researchers.

Writing a research proposal

Often, writing a research proposal is an assessment requirement for undergraduate or postgraduate research students. While this may feel an onerous task, the ability to write a research proposal is important for any nurse or midwife. For example, you may want to conduct a small study in your clinical workplace for which approval needs to be sought or for which you require funding, or you may want to undertake a study as part of a research degree. Strong research proposals are important in the wider competitive area of funding applications. For all of these situations, a research proposal precedes embarking on the study.

research proposal
a structured blueprint for a proposed study

A research proposal is a blueprint for a planned study. It outlines the background, design, methods and significance of the research. In a competitive environment, a high-quality research proposal can optimise the likelihood of success and ensure a well-managed project that reaches completion. It is important, then, for the proposal to be developed carefully and structured in a logical way. In this section, we will work through the key aspects of writing a high-quality research proposal.

Title

The proposal should begin with a title. This should be clear and concise, so a reader will know exactly what the proposed study is about. Sometimes, the title also contains the type of study being proposed.

Abstract

The abstract presents a brief summary of the proposed research. While it usually appears early in the proposal, it is common for this part to be written after the rest of the proposal has been developed. In general, the abstract should not be more than 300 words in length. It should cover the following information:

- brief background to the proposed study
- aim of the research
- methodology and design for the study
- location of the study

- participants in the study
- data collection, management and analysis approaches
- potential uses for the findings.

Introduction and background

This section should clearly convey to the reader the key focus of your research study and why it is an important study to do. This section should provide a basic introduction to the reader of what your topic is about and the reasons for doing the study. While it may be perfectly clear to you, the reader of your proposal may not be at all familiar with the topic, so this is particularly important if you do not want to lose their interest early on.

Study significance

It is here that you need to demonstrate why your study is necessary and what benefits it will produce. It needs to convince the reader that the study is required and say how the findings will make an impact. It may also be called the *rationale* or *justification* for the study—that is, the reason for the study to be conducted.

Literature review

The literature review provides an overview of the current state of knowledge in your topic. It should provide a summary and a critique of existing research. The idea is to demonstrate a gap in what is currently known, to further justify the need for the study and for your findings, which will fill that gap. The literature review should discuss research no more than five years old to demonstrate the gap in present knowledge. If critical information exists that is older than five years, it should be presented in the background section.

Research problem, aim and question

This section needs to identify the problem to be addressed by the proposed research. The aim of the research is presented as a broad, overarching statement about what the study will set out to do. It is followed by the research question and, in the case of quantitative research, a hypothesis (see Chapter 4).

The research question must be clearly articulated, as it will guide the whole research, and it needs to be written as a question that your research sets out to answer. It is crucial for the research question to be constructed in such a way that it is answerable and realistically able to be researched. In some studies, there will be one main overarching research question which is subdivided into a number of further questions.

Theoretical framework

The theoretical, or conceptual, framework underpinning your research is important. It demonstrates how you are planning to approach the research from a theoretical or philosophical (methodological) position. This is important, as it will guide your research design, data collection and analysis. For example, if you are proposing to do qualitative research, your theoretical framework might be informed by phenomenology or grounded theory. This section may also be conceptually driven, being underpinned by a philosophical position. Whatever your position, it needs to be clearly outlined. This is particularly important when the proposal is being written for academic purposes.

Research design

The research design presents the practicalities of the actual research and constitutes the largest component of the proposal. It should provide a step-by-step description of how the research will actually be carried out. The steps need to align directly with the research aim, research question and theoretical framework. There are numerous categories of information needed here, which are discussed below.

Methods

The methods are the approaches that will be taken to allow the research question to be answered. For example, you might use survey design, semi-structured interviews or observation. There may also be different phases to your study if you are using mixed methods approaches.

Participants

It is essential to identify who the participants will be in your proposed study. There are several questions that need to be answered in doing this:

- What will be the participants' particular characteristics?
- How will participants be invited to participate?
- How will they be recruited, and by whom?
- How many participants will be needed?
- Will there be inclusion and exclusion criteria?
- Are they likely to be a vulnerable group? If so, who will need to be involved to ensure they are protected during the research?

Data collection

It is necessary to clarify the nature of the data collection to be employed. Again, it is useful to consider the following:

- Where will the data be collected?
- Who will collect the data?
- How long will the data collection take?

Instruments

The tools you plan to use need to be clearly explained; for example:

- What data collection instruments will be used?
- If they are questionnaires, have they been previously used and shown they are valid and reliable
- If they are qualitative interviews, what questions are to be asked of participants?

In the case of questionnaires, if they have not been validated previously, a pilot study may be needed before the actual study commences, in order for this to be done.

Data management and analysis

How you plan to handle the data when you have them needs to be clearly described. If you will be using quantitative data, this might include information about organising and cleaning up data and entering data into computer programs, along with descriptions of the tests you plan to run. If you will be using qualitative data, you will likely be employing a form of content or thematic analysis, for which there are many approaches, so you will need to describe the steps involved. This includes steps you will take to ensure your interpretations are accurate. Some aspects to consider here include:

- What processes will be used for data management?
- Will data be entered into a particular software program?
- How will the data be analysed?
- What tests will be conducted?
- If qualitative data will be collected, how will these be analysed?
- How will rigour in data analysis be achieved? (This is particularly important in qualitative research.)

Ethical considerations

This is a very important section. You need to identify who is required to approve the study, such as hospital managers. If the study will involve people, it will also require the approval of at least one Human Research Ethics Committee. If you are studying at a university and doing clinical research, it is likely that you will need approval from both the university and the hospital. If you are doing a multi-centre study, you may require even more approvals.

This section also needs to clearly outline all of the potential ethical issues involved in the conduct of the research. (We covered this in detail in Chapter 7.) It is particularly important to ensure that in your proposal you include the steps you will take to protect the rights of people who are participating in your research.

Timeline

There needs to be a clearly outlined timeline that demonstrates the different activities of the study and when they will occur. It should clearly show the length of the project and when each activity will begin and end. This is an important component for demonstrating that the proposed study is feasible within the suggested timeframe. Often, this information is presented in a visual format in a chart or table.

Budget and resources

Regardless of whether you are formally seeking funding or not, carefully consider how much your proposed study will cost and what resources will be needed to successfully complete it. It is also important in this section to justify why each item is necessary for your project. The budget should be realistic, with accurate and defendable calculations, including other costs such as charges from the university for office space or other organisation-imposed overheads. The types of items to consider here are listed below, followed by examples:

- **Personnel costs** Staff to be employed on the project, such as research assistants
- **Equipment** Digital recorder for qualitative interviews
- **Services** Transcription of qualitative interviews
- **Printing** Questionnaires, consent forms, final reports
- **Travel** Transport to visit participants, usually as costs per kilometre
- **Catering** Afternoon tea for focus group participants
- **Room hire** Daily room hire for conducting focus groups
- **Dissemination costs** Travel to, registration and accommodation for conference attendance to present findings
- **In-kind contributions** Equivalent costs for items, such as personnel, that are to be provided free of charge.

Research team

If you propose to lead a team-based project, you will need to provide information on each team member, such as:

- their qualifications and professional affiliations
- the expertise and previous experience each brings to the research
- their individual roles in the project.

Dissemination plan

It is useless to do any research without disseminating its findings, so that others can apply them to their own contexts. A research proposal should always include a plan for how the findings will be communicated to others. This might include:

- peer-reviewed international journals, with suggestions of the most relevant journals
- national or international conference presentations, with suggestions of relevant conferences
- distribution to funding or other professional bodies
- circulation through social media.

References

This should contain all of the primary sources used in the proposal.

Appendices

Any supplementary documentation should be presented as appendices. This might include such things as questionnaires, ethical approvals obtained, letters of support and curricula vitae of the researchers.

RESEARCH EXAMPLE 10.3 A nursing research proposal

In our case study, Angela has completed her clinical research nurse role and has decided she would like to conduct her own research studies through enrolling in a doctor of philosophy. Her previous research work has sparked an interest in menopause, particularly the experiences of young women having to cope with early menopause. As part of her degree application, she needs to write a proposal. This is what she produces:

Title Young immigrant women's lived experience of early menopause: A phenomenological study

Background Early onset, or premature, menopause is defined as being the onset of menopause prior to the age of 40 years. Besides leading to fertility issues, early menopause can cause a range of medical and psychological issues that necessitate health professional attention. Women experiencing this condition require individualised hormone therapy and counselling (Faubion et al. 2015). Little is known about the experiences of immigrant women experiencing early onset menopause, particularly whether they seek assistance for such issues and whether the existing support mechanisms meet their needs. In addition, it is unclear if there are additional cultural factors that impact on their experience of the condition.

Study significance Early onset menopause is a challenging condition. However, little is known specifically about the experiences of immigrant women with the condition. This study will provide understandings of the issues faced by immigrant women experiencing early menopause so that specifically tailored support and care can be developed.

Literature review The absence of oestrogen caused by early onset menopause can lead to a range of long-term health effects, including cardiovascular disease, neurological disease, osteoporosis, mood, sexual and psychological disorders and premature death (Shuster et al. 2010). A study by Strezova et al. (2017) found that cultural factors influenced the perceptions and experiences of menopause in Macedonian women living in Australia. However, little recent literature could be sourced relating to other immigrant groups. No studies could be sourced that have specifically examined the experiences of immigrant women who have undergone early onset menopause.

Research aim To explore the lived experiences of immigrant women impacted by early onset menopause.

Research question What are the lived experiences of immigrant women with early onset (premature) menopause?

Theoretical framework Phenomenology will underpin the study. This approach aims to reflect the lived experiences of participants and has a long tradition through many philosophers. This research will employ van Manen's (1990) hermeneutic phenomenology. It is a practical approach and allows for insights to be drawn out, along with the meanings and understandings that participants give to their experiences.

Research design Semi-structured interviews will be conducted with approximately fifteen to twenty immigrant women, aged in their twenties or thirties, who have experienced early onset menopause. Women will be recruited by social media (for example, Facebook) and snowball sampling. An interview guide will be developed to guide the interviews. Interviews will be conducted by the student researcher in a quiet and mutually agreed place. Data will be analysed using thematic analysis informed by the work of Braun and Clark (2006). Themes will be reviewed for accuracy by the research supervisors.

Ethical considerations Women will be provided with verbal information about the study and provide written informed consent prior to undertaking the interview. Confidentiality will be maintained through the use of pseudonyms in reporting the findings. Prior to the interviews, ethical approval to conduct the study will be sought from the university Human Research Ethics Committee.

Timeline

Year 1

January–June Undertake a detailed literature review to inform the study

July–September Refine study, develop interview schedule

October–December Seek ethical approval

Year 2

January–July Recruit participants and conduct interviews

August–December Conduct data analysis

Year 3

January–June Write chapters

July–December Finalise thesis for submission

Budget No funding will be sought for this study. The student researcher will transcribe the interviews.

References

Braun, V. & Clarke, V., 2006, 'Using thematic analysis in psychology', *Qualitative Research in Psychology*, vol. 3, no. 2, pp. 77–101.

Faubion, S.S., Kuhle, C.L., Shuster, L.T. & Rocca, W.A., 2015, 'Long-term health consequences of premature or early menopause and considerations for management', *Climacteric*, vol. 18, no. 4, pp. 483–491.

Shuster, L.T., Rhodes, D.J., Gostout, B.S., Grossardt, B.R. & Rocca, W.A., 2010, 'Premature menopause or early menopause: Long-term health consequences', *Maturitas*, vol. 65, no. 2, p. 161–166.

Strezova, A., O'Neill, S., O'Callaghan, C., Perry, A., Liu, J. & Eden, J., 2017, 'Cultural issues in menopause: An exploratory qualitative study of Macedonian women in Australia', *Menopause*, vol. 24, no. 3, pp. 308–315.

van Manen, M., 1990, *Researching Lived Experience: Human science for an action sensitive pedagogy*, Albany: State University of New York Press.

Questions for consideration

- Is Angela's research aim clear?
- Is the research methodology appropriate to the study aim?
- Is the scope of the proposed research activity clear and well outlined?
- Are the proposed data collection and analysis processes appropriate to the chosen methodology?
- Is the timeline for the study realistic?
- Are there aspects that could be further elaborated?

Additional hints for writing a research proposal

While we have covered the key elements of the research proposal, there are also some helpful hints we suggest you consider before submitting your proposal:

- Remember you are trying to impress the reader, especially if you are seeking funding! Ensure that your proposal looks professional in its appearance and that spelling, grammar and layout are all perfect.
- Ask someone who is unfamiliar with your topic to review the proposal. It needs to sound logical and understandable to someone who does not know the topic as well as you.
- Avoid the use of acronyms. While you know what they mean, the reader may not, and an acronym may mean different things to different people, depending on their context; for example, *PE* may mean *pulmonary embolism* to a nurse but *pre-eclampsia* to a midwife.
- If you are seeking funding, closely review the proposal requirements of the funding agency. Each agency has specific and different requirements.

ACTIVITY 10.4 Developing a research proposal

Using the research proposal framework provided in the previous section, begin to develop a proposal for a research study that you could undertake.
- What aspects of developing the proposal are particularly challenging?
- Where might you be able to go for support in further developing your proposal?

CHAPTER SUMMARY

Nurses and midwives have increasing opportunities to take on research-focused roles, engaging in the generation of new knowledge to support nursing, midwifery and health care more generally. A variety of research-based courses is available to arm students with the skills needed to engage in research-focused roles, and we have explored many of these in this chapter. The ability to write a quality research proposal is important for nurses and midwives, whether they are engaged in clinical or academic work. We have explored the key components of such a proposal and what each should contain.

CHAPTER REVIEW QUESTIONS

- What is a clinical trial?
- What research roles are available for nurses and midwives? How do they differ?
- What pathways can nurses and midwives take to pursue research activities?
- Where can nurses and midwives seek funding to support their research?
- What are the key aspects to developing a quality research proposal?

QUESTIONS FOR DISCUSSION

- How can nurses and midwives contribute to the generation of research?
- Why should nurses and midwives engage in research activities?
- What are the pathways for nurses and midwives to pursue their research interests?
- What benefits and challenges might be faced by nurses and midwives engaging in research activities?

QUESTIONS FOR PERSONAL REFLECTION

- How has your learning in this chapter influenced your perception of research roles in nursing or midwifery?
- Would you consider a future research career? If so, how might you get there?

USEFUL WEB RESOURCES

Australian Research Council <www.arc.gov.au>

International Network for Doctoral Education in Nursing <https://nursing.jhu.edu/excellence/inden/index.html>

National Health and Medical Research Council <www.nhmrc.gov.au>

REFERENCES AND FURTHER READING

Barker, L., Rattihalli, R.R. & Field, D., 2015, 'How to write a good research grant proposal', *Paediatrics and Child Health*, vol. 26, no. 3, pp. 105–109.

Blanco, M.A. & Lee, M.Y., 2012, 'Twelve tips for writing educational research grant proposals', *Medical Teacher*, vol. 34, pp. 450–453.

Bowrey, S. & Thompson, J.P., 2014, 'Nursing research: Ethics, consent and good practice', *Nursing Times*, vol. 110, no. 1/3, pp. 20–23.

Clarke, S.P., 2016, 'Navigating a research-focused doctoral program in nursing', *Nursing Management*, vol. 47, no. 1, pp. 19–20.

Cleland, V., 2012, 'Nursing research and graduate education', *Nursing Outlook*, vol. 60, pp. 259–263.

Cronenwett, L., Dracup, K., Grey, M., McCauley, L., Meleis, A. & Salmon, M., 2011, 'The doctor of nursing practice: A national workforce perspective', *Nursing Outlook*, vol. 59, pp. 9–17.

Edwardson, S.R., 2010, 'Doctor of philosophy and doctor of nursing practice as complementary degrees', *Journal of Professional Nursing*, vol. 26, no. 3, pp. 137–140.

Florczak, K.L., Poradzisz, M. & Kostovich, C., 2014, 'Traditional or translational research for nursing: More PhDs please', *Nursing Science Quarterly*, vol. 27, no. 3, pp. 195–200.

Halcomb, E., Smyth, E., Moxham, L., Traynor, V. & Fernandez, R., 2018, 'Bachelor of nursing programs in Australia: Trends and key challenges', *Collegian*, doi: 10.1016/j.colegn.2017.11.003.

Hollins, C.J. & Fleming, V., 2010, 'A 15-step model for writing a research proposal', *British Journal of Midwifery*, vol. 18, no. 12, pp. 791–798.

Jones, H.C., 2015, 'Clinical research nurse or nurse researcher?', *Nursing Times*, vol. 111, no. 19, pp. 12–14.

Kivunja, C., 2016, 'How to write an effective research proposal for higher degree research in higher education: Lessons from practice', *International Journal of Higher Education*, vol. 5, no. 2, pp. 163–172.

Klopper, H., 2008, 'The qualitative research proposal', *Curationis*, vol. 31, no. 4, pp. 62–72.

Kunhunny, S. & Salmon, D., 2017, 'The evolving professional identity of the clinical research nurse: A qualitative exploration', *Journal of Clinical Nursing*, vol. 26, pp. 5121–5132.

Marshall, L.S., 2012, 'Research commentary: Grant writing', part 1: 'First things first …', *Journal of Radiology Nursing*, vol. 31, no. 4, pp. 154–155.

Marshall, L.S., 2013, 'Research commentary: Grant writing', part 2: 'Application/proposal components', *Journal of Radiology Nursing*, vol. 32, no. 1, pp. 48–51.

Rattihalli, R.R. & Field, D.J., 2011, 'How to write a good research grant proposal', *Paediatrics and Child Health*, vol. 22, no. 2, pp. 57–60.

Rodrigo, P., 2013, 'Could you be a research nurse?', *Nursing Standard*, vol. 27, no. 44, pp. 62–63.

Seeman, E., 2015, 'The ABC of writing a grant proposal', *Osteoporosis International*, vol. 26, pp. 1665–1666.

Watmough, S., Flynn, M., Wright, A. & Fry, K., 2010, 'Research nurse or nurse researcher?', *British Journal of Cardiac Nursing*, vol. 5, no. 8, pp. 396–399.

Wilkes, L., Jackson, D., Miranda, C. & Watson, R., 2012, 'The role of clinical trial nurses: An Australian perspective', *Collegian*, vol. 19, pp. 239–246.

GLOSSARY OF TERMS

abstract   a summary of a published article or a conference presentation

action research   a cyclical research approach designed to facilitate change through empowering participants

AGREE   a study reporting guideline for clinical practice guidelines

analysis of variance   a statistical test used for comparing a continuous (ratio or interval) variable between three or more groups; also known as ANOVA

anonymity   the state of a research participant's identity being unknown to researchers

autonomy   the right to exercise one's will

beneficence   to do good; in research, a study should aim to have good potential outcomes

bias   a systematic error in the way participants are selected, outcomes are measured or data are analysed that leads to results being inaccurate

blinding or **masking**   concealment of group allocation from study participants, researchers, others involved in the research, or all three

Boolean operator   a term used to combine keywords or search results in specific ways; terms available are *AND*, *OR* and *NOT*

CARE   a study reporting guideline for case reports

case-control design   a non-experimental study design where a group of participants with a certain condition (cases) is studied alongside a similar group of people without the condition (control)

case study   a research approach that examines the complexities of unique stories to explore a particular phenomenon

categorical or **nominal data**   values that represent a classification or group membership—for example, gender and hair colour

central tendency   a measure, generally towards the middle of a dataset, around which data points are clustered; potential measures are mean, median and mode

CHEERS   a reporting standard for economic evaluations

chi square   a statistical test used for comparing two categorical variables, each of which has two or more values

clinical audit   a review of current practice and performance against best available evidence

clinical doctorate   a clinically focused doctoral degree

clinical practice guidelines   guidelines for informing clinical practice developed from best available evidence

clinical trial   a study that examines the effectiveness of new treatments in clinical practice with a view to enhancing or changing the management of patients

cluster random sampling   a study sampling where selection of participants is by groups rather than individuals

cluster randomised controlled trial   a randomised controlled trial where the unit of randomisation is not the individual participant but a group of participants

coding   a process of marking keywords or phrases in text

coercion   the unethical process of pressurising someone to participate in research

cohort design   a non-experimental study design where participants (the cohort) are studied over a period of time

confidence intervals   parameters between which the true difference between measurements, or effect of an intervention, would lie if it were measured in the whole population

confidentiality   the protection of information that a research participant does not wish to be made public; this can include, but is not limited to, concealment of their identity

confirmability   the degree to which qualitative findings represent participants' perspectives

confounder   a factor not related to an intervention that can influence the outcome being studied

CONSORT   a reporting standard for randomised controlled trials

contamination   a situation where members of a study control group are exposed to the intervention

content analysis   a deductive process of analysing qualitative data; it can be done numerically or in categories

convenience sampling a sampling method where people are approached because they are readily accessible, and they self-select to take part

correlation a statistical test used for comparing two continuous variables when both are measured, not manipulated

correlational design a non-experimental study design in which the aim is to investigate associations between the outcome of interest and other factors

credibility ensuring interpretations and conclusions drawn from data are truly reflective

Critical Appraisal Skills Programme a tool for evaluating research quality; also known as CASP

critique assessment of a research study to identify strengths, weaknesses and quality

cross-sectional design a non-experimental study design where data are collected at one specific point in time

data information collected to answer a research question

data analysis the process of analysing collected data to draw conclusions

data collection the process of collecting data to answer a research question

data extraction the process of selecting data from studies for inclusion in a systematic or scoping review

data immersion the process by which the qualitative researcher absorbs themselves in data to extract content and meanings

data saturation the point in qualitative data collection where no new data are being obtained

Declaration of Helsinki a set of ethical research principles for human research developed by the World Medical Association

deductive approach a research approach involving developing and testing a hypothesis

deferred or **retrospective consent** formal consent for data to be used after those data have been collected

dependability the consistency of qualitative findings in other, similar conditions

dependent variable the outcome of interest in a quantitative study

descriptive qualitative research a qualitative research approach that seeks to describe a particular phenomenon

descriptive quantitative design   a non-experimental quantitative study design in which the aim is to describe and quantify a concept of interest; sometimes called an exploratory design

descriptive statistics   measures used to summarise raw data

direct quotation   text taken word-for-word from another person's work; this requires the inclusion of quotation marks citation and possibly also the page number of the work from which the words were taken

discourse analysis   a research approach that examines social and political factors that shape the development of certain practices or circumstances

dispersion   a measure of the degree of variability in a dataset; potential measures are variance, standard deviation, range, interquartile range and frequency

dissemination   communication of research findings, for example, through publication or presentation

EQUATOR Network   Enhancing the Quality and Transparency of Health Research Network

ethical approval   a part of the research process that involves seeking formal approval from a Human Research Ethics Committee to conduct a study

ethics   a discipline area concerned with moral values and conduct

ethnography   a research approach that examines cultural patterns existing in a particular group

ethnomethodology   a research approach that examines the ways in which people feel, understand and explain their world

evidence   knowledge derived from systematic research

evidence-based practice   practice informed by best available research evidence, clinical expertise and client preference

exclusion criteria   characteristics that exclude a participant from a study or a study from a review

external validity   the ability to generalise the results of a study beyond the study sample

fittingness or **transferability**   the capacity for conclusions from qualitative research to have similar meanings to other, similar populations

focus group   a group of people with which an interview is conducted at the same time

frequency   the count of the occurrences of values in a dataset expressed as a number, a percentage or a proportion

grey literature   literature not published in academic sources

grounded theory   a research methodology that examines social processes in order to develop theory

H-index   a measure of a researcher's publication citations

handsearching   manual searching for literature for inclusion in a literature review

hierarchy of evidence   levels of authority attributed to different forms of research evidence

historical research   a research approach that examines the historical development of a particular concept or situation

honours degree   an undergraduate research degree, usually comprising one year of full-time-equivalent study

HREC *see* Human Research Ethics Committee

Human Research Ethics Committee   a committee that oversees compliance of human research with ethical standards; also known as an HREC

hypothesis   a statement about assumed variable relationships that can be tested

impact factor   a measure of the impact of a journal, relating to citations of the papers that it publishes

implementation science   an emerging scientific field examining implementation of existing evidence into practice and policy

implied consent   agreement to take part can be assumed by an activity, such as filling out a questionnaire

inclusion criteria   characteristics that a potential participant or a study must possess to be included in research or a literature review

independent variable   a specific factor that could influence the study outcome

inductive approach   an interpretive approach that seeks to develop a new theory or model from data, moving from specific observations to make generalisations

inferential statistics   tests carried out on data to determine whether the results can be generalised from the sample to the population

informed consent   a person's agreement to be included in research based on full disclosure of what is involved

internal validity   the ability to attribute the outcome of a research study to the effect of the independent variable and not some other factor

interpretive research   qualitative research that seeks to make meaning of a phenomenon

interquartile range   the difference between the 1st and 3rd quartiles; also known as IQR

interval data   values between which distances (intervals) correspond to real, meaningful, consistent differences in the phenomenon being measured—for example, temperature

intervention   a procedure to which research participants are exposed by the researchers rather than by their own choice; the procedure is managed and controlled by the researchers

interview   a method of data collection where data are collected verbally

interview schedule   key questions used for guiding a research interview

justice   the fair treatment of research participants

knowledge translation   the process of translating research knowledge into practice contexts

Likert scale   a rating scale that allows participants to indicate their level of agreement with presented statements

literature review   a synthesis of previously published research conducted on a particular topic

masking *see* blinding or masking

mean   the average of a set of numbers, obtained by summing all the values and dividing by the number of values in the dataset

median   the middle value when the values in a dataset are placed in numerical order; if there is an even number of values, the median is calculated by taking the average of the two middle numbers

Medical Subject Headings   a thesaurus of terms maintained by the US National Library of Medicine; also known as MeSH

member checking   the process of returning to participants to check interpretations made

MeSH *see* Medical Subject Headings

methodology   the philosophical beliefs or assumptions that influence a study's design

midwife researcher   a midwife who conducts research

mixed methods   a research approach involving mixing of more than one research method in one study, usually combining quantitative and qualitative approaches

mode   the most frequently occurring value in a dataset

narrative research   a research approach that explores the experiences of people through the stories they tell

narrative review *see* traditional narrative review

nominal data *see* categorical or nominal data

non-maleficence   to do no harm; in research, a study should not cause harm to participants

non-probability sampling   sampling that does not involve random selection

normal distribution   symmetrical distribution of data with the majority of data points clustered around the centre; when represented graphically it forms a bell-shaped curve

Nuremberg Code   a set of ethical research principles developed in response to human experimentation during the Second World War

nurse researcher   a nurse who conducts research

observation   a data collection method where participants are observed in a specific context

opt out consent   a mechanism whereby people refuse consent to take part in research, or for information about them to be used in research, before they become eligible for inclusion; if they do not take up this option they will be included automatically

ordinal data   values that are ordered (ranked), but between which the differences cannot be quantified

paradigm   a particular viewpoint of the world

paraphrasing   rewriting ideas in one's own words

participant observation   a data collection method where participants are observed in a specific context

participatory research   qualitative research that actively involves participants in making change

peer review   the process of evaluating an article for its suitability for publication. It is usually undertaken by a minimum of two people with expertise in the topic, the methods used, or both

percentile   the value at or below which lies a certain percentage of values in a distribution

person-centred care   care that is focused on the person and in which the person is given autonomy to make decisions about their care

phenomenology   a qualitative research methodology that examines human lived experience

photovoice   a qualitative research approach using photographs to present viewpoints from participants' unique worlds

PICO   an acronym used to name the key aspects of a systematic review, usually referring to *population*, *intervention*, *comparator* and *outcome*

population   the entire group of people to whom researchers want to apply their findings

power   the likelihood of a test correctly indicating a real effect of an intervention due to sufficient sample size

pre-post test   a study design where measurements are performed before and after an intervention

predatory journal   a non-credible journal that exploits researchers by charging publication fees without providing academic oversight and rigour, such as peer review

primary source   a paper that provides first-hand reporting of a study by the researcher

probability   the likelihood of a result occurring by chance

probability sampling   sampling based on random selection

protocol *see* review protocol

purposive sampling   a sampling approach involving purposefully selecting research participants

qualitative descriptive research   a qualitative research approach that seeks to describe a particular phenomenon

qualitative research   a research approach, primarily inductive, that seeks to make meaning of human experience

quantitative research   a research approach, largely deductive, that emphasises objective measurement of information and its numerical analysis

quartile ranking   ranking of journals into four categories, where the 1st quartile, or top 25 per cent (Q1), contains the highest-ranking journals

quasi-experimental design   an experimental study design where there is no control group, or allocation is not performed randomly

quota sampling   study sampling where participants are selected until the quota is filled

randomised controlled trial or **true experiment**   research design that is the most reliable in establishing cause-and-effect relationships, requiring the presence of an intervention, a control group, and random allocation to the experimental and the control groups; also known as RCT

range   the difference between the highest and lowest value in a dataset

ratio data   values between which the distances are meaningful and consistent; these variables have a *natural zero*, indicating possible absence of the entity (for example, length, duration, weight), and can be multiplied and divided

RCT *see* randomised controlled trial or true experiment

realist evaluation   an approach to evaluating programs and how they work

regression   a statistical test examining the effect of manipulating one continuous variable (the independent variable) on a continuous outcome variable (the dependent variable)

reliability   the consistency with which a research instrument measures the construct

research aim   what a researcher is seeking to achieve by doing a study

research degree   a degree that entails conducting a research study

research integrity   honesty in research conduct and reporting

research merit   an ethical principle requiring that a research study must have potential benefit and that this benefit can be realised

research midwife   a midwife who works with a team on a clinical trial

research nurse   a nurse who works with a team on a clinical trial

research process   the whole process of conducting research, from the original idea to the dissemination of findings

research proposal   a structured blueprint for a proposed study

research question   the question that a research study is designed to answer

retrospective consent *see* deferred or retrospective consent

review protocol   a detailed plan for undertaking a systematic or scoping review

sample   the subset of a population selected to take part in the research

sampling   the process of selecting research participants

saturation *see* data saturation

scoping review   a structured literature review that employs a protocol to explore a broad topic area, sometimes to identify gaps in what is known

secondary source   a paper that reports on someone else's research study

self-determination   the freedom to make one's own decisions

simple random sampling   a sampling method where a random-number generator is used to select the required number of study participants from a population

skewed distribution   asymmetrical data distribution; when represented graphically the curve has a longer tail at one end than the other

snowball sampling   a sampling method where current participants in a study recommend future potential participants

SQUIRE   a reporting standard for quality improvement studies

SRQR   a reporting standard for qualitative research

standard deviation   the square root of the variance, in essence correcting for the squaring of values that occurred in calculating the variance; it is nearly always used in preference to the variance

STARD   a reporting standard for diagnostic and prognostic studies

stratified random sampling   a sampling method where the population is divided according to one or more characteristics and a random sample is drawn from each

STROBE   a reporting standard for observational studies

systematic review a literature review that uses a structured question and search approach along with critical appraisal and quality analysis of studies

systematic sampling a sampling method where participants are chosen not at random but according to a specific schedule

t-test a statistical test used for comparing a continuous (ratio or interval) variable between two groups

thematic analysis an interpretive process of organising qualitative data into themes

theme a grouping of data containing similar meanings; it emerges through thematic analysis

theoretical sampling a sampling technique used in grounded theory, involving sampling until the generated theory is complete

traditional narrative review a subjective, non-critical review of the literature where included research is selected by the author

transferability *see* fittingness or transferability

triangulation the use of multiple methods or data sources that the researcher can verify and from which they can draw accurate conclusions

true experiment *see* randomised controlled trial or true experiment

truncator a symbol used at the end of part of a word in a database search to enable searching for all words that begin with the same letters

trustworthiness the attribute of rigour in qualitative research

validity of an instrument the accuracy with which a research instrument or tool measures what it is supposed to measure

variable any measured concept or characteristic that can vary in a study

variance the average of the differences between each individual value and the mean

wildcard a symbol used in place of a single letter to enable database searching for all variations of spelling

INDEX